CONTROVERSIES IN RHEUMATOLOGY

CONTROVERSIES IN RHEUMATOLOGY

Edited by

DAVID A ISENBERG MD, FRCP
Centre for Rheumatology/Bloomsbury
Rheumatology Unit
Department of Medicine
University College London
London, UK

LORI B TUCKER, MD
Department of Pediatric Rheumatology
Floating Hospital for Infants and Children
New England Medical Center
Boston, USA

MARTIN DUNITZ

First published in the United Kingdom in 1997 by
Martin Dunitz Ltd
The Livery House
7–9 Pratt Street
London NW1 0AE

A CIP catalogue record for this book is available from the British Library

ISBN 1-85317-395-9

Composition by Scribe Design, Gillingham, Kent
Printed and bound in Great Britain by Biddles Ltd, Guildford and King's Lynn

Contents

Preface

As clinical medical students we tend to be taught in shades of white or black, thus: 'The antibiotic is to be given in four doses per day for five days only...' or 'Drug X is completely contraindicated if the patient is in renal failure'. In reality of course there are many grey areas in clinical medicine, some of which stimulate major differences of opinion. From these more controversial areas we have selected 15 topics covering a range of adult and paediatric rheumatological conundrums for critical review and assessment.

Our topic list is not exhaustive and editorial licence has been allowed in choosing a range of issues that we think are of general concern and/or of particular interest to us. Nevertheless we hope the reader will appreciate the broad, if eclectic, scope of the subjects chosen. The authors, whom we acknowledge gratefully for their ability (in the main!) to meet the tight deadlines given, have taken up our challenge to review the conflicting data dispassionately and not to be afraid of expressing their opinions.

We cannot claim to have resolved the controversies, but hope that the chapters will contribute to the ongoing debate in these problem areas and help the reader make up his/her mind about a range of controversial contemporary issues in clinical rheumatology.

David A Isenberg
London
Lori B Tucker
Boston

Acknowledgements

We wish to thank Ann Maitland for much of the organizational work and secretarial support that went into the production of this volume. We also thank Lee Nelson for reviewing one of the chapters for us, and Lionel Joseph and Buzzy Olin for their support at an important time.

Contributors

Bernard Amor, MD
Rheumatology Department
Hôpital Cochin
27 rue du faubourg Saint Jacques
75679 Paris Cedex 14
FRANCE

Peter Brooks, MD, FRACP
Medical Professorial Unit
St Vincent's Hospital
Darlinghurst
Sydney 2010
AUSTRALIA

Gerd-R Burmester, MD
Department of Rheumatology and
Clinical Immunology
Charité University Hospital
Humboldt Univeristy
D-10098 Berlin
GERMANY

James T Cassidy, MD
Department of Child Health
University of Missouri
One Hospital Drive
Columbia MO 65212
USA

Ernest H C Choy, MD, MRCP
Rheumatology Unit
Division of Medicine
Guy's Hospital UMDS
London SE1 9RT
UK

Ali Hajeer, PhD
ARC Epidemiology Research Unit
University of Manchester
Oxford Road
Manchester, M13 9PT
UK

Philip J Hashkes, MD
Children's Hospital Medical Center
Division of Pediatric Rheumatology
3333 Burnet Avenue
Cincinnati OH 45299-3039
USA

David A Isenberg, MD, FRCP
Professor of Rheumatology
Bloomsbury Rheumatology Unit
University College London
London, W1P 9PG
UK

Thomas Kamradt, MD
Department of Rheumatology
and Clinical Immunology
Charité University Hospital
Humboldt Univeristy
D-10098 Berlin
GERMANY

Gabrielle H Kingsley, FRCP
Rheumatology Unit
Guy's and St Thomas's
Medical and Dental School
Division of Medicine
Guy's Hospital
London SE1 9RT
UK

Andreas Krause, MD
Department of Rheumatology
and Clinical Immunology
Charité University Hospital
Humboldt Univeristy
D-10098 Berlin
GERMANY

Gavin Lee, MBBS, MRCP
Rheumatology Fellow
Department of Medicine
Queen Mary Hospital
HONG KONG

Daniel J Lovell, MD, MPH
Children's Hospital Medical Center
Division of Pediatric Rheumatology
3333 Burnet Avenue
Cincinnati OH 45299-3039
USA

Clare E McLure, MRCP
Bloomsbury Rheumatology Unit
University College Hospital
London
W1P 9PG
UK

Ola Nived, MD, PhD
Associate Professor and Chairman
Department of Rheumatology
University Hospital
S-22185 Lund
SWEDEN

William E R Ollier, PhD
ARC Epidemiology Research Unit
University of Manchester
Oxford Road
Manchester
M13 9PT
UK

Gabriel S Panayi, MD, DSC, FRCP
Rheumatology Unit
Guy's and St Thomas's
Medical and Dental School
Division of Medicine
Guy's Hospital
London SE1 9RT
UK

Michael Shipley, MA, MD, FRCP
Clinical Director
Bloomsbury Rheumatology Unit
University College London
London
W1P 9PG
UK

Roger Smith, MD, PhD, FRCP
Nuffield Orthopaedic Centre
Headington
Oxford
OX3 7LD
UK

Taunton R Southwood, FRCP
Department of Rheumatology
Faculty of Medicine and Dentistry
University of Birmingham
Edgbaston, Birmingham
B15 2TT
UK

Gunnar Sturfelt, MD
Associate Professor
Department of Rheumatology
University Hospital Lund
S-22185 Lund
SWEDEN

Roger D Sturrock, MD, FRCP
Centre for Rheumatic Diseases
Glasgow Royal Infirmary
Glasgow
G31 2ER
UK

Antoine Toubert, MD
INSERM U 386
15 rue de l'Ecole de Médecine
75006 Paris
FRANCE

Lori B Tucker, MD
Pediatric Rheumatology
Floating Hospital
for Infants & Children
New England Medical Center
Boston MA 02111
USA

Frank H J van den Hoogen, MD
Rheumatology Department
University Hospital Nijmegen
6500 HB Nijmegen
THE NETHERLANDS

Leo B A van de Putte, MD
Rheumatology Department
University Hospital Nijmegen
6500 HB Nijmegen
THE NETHERLANDS

1

Does the HLA-DRB1 shared epitope really contribute that much to the development or severity of rheumatoid arthritis?

William ER Ollier, Ali Hajeer

RA has a genetic basis

Rheumatoid arthritis (RA) is a complex disease and twin studies clearly demonstrate that both genetic and environmental factors play a significant role in disease aetiology.[1,2] An important step towards clarifying the genetic component came from the gradual realization that HLA-DR4 was strongly associated with RA risk.[3,4] However, a better appreciation of the complexity of RA aetiology has been gained from calculations indicating that HLA only accounts for one-third to one-half of the total genetic contribution,[5] suggesting that whilst HLA is likely to be the major RA susceptibility locus, other genes also contribute to susceptibility and clinical expression. This is in keeping with the clinical heterogeneity observed in RA in terms of age of onset, range of severity, and rate of progression.

Table 1.1 Association of rheumatoid arthritis with HLA-DRB1 alleles other than HLA-DR4

Population	HLA-DRB1 allele	References
Asian Indian	*0101, *1001	8,9
Native N. American	*1402	10
Greek	*0101, *1001	11,12
Spanish	*0101, *1001	13,14
Basque	*0101, *1001	15
Israeli	*0101, *1001	16,17
Zimbabwean	*1001	18
Zulu	*1001	19

RA is associated with multiple HLA types

The association of HLA with RA was initially explained either as DR4 being an RA disease susceptibility (DS) gene or as DR4 acting as a marker allele in linkage disequilibrium with a DS gene. As more information became available about HLA, several pertinent facts emerged. Firstly, it was realized that HLA-DR types were only broad serological definitions, and examination at the DNA sequence level revealed that some alleles of the DRB1 gene could not be discriminated from each other by antibodies used in tissue typing. Secondly, a large number of 'DR4-related' DRB1 alleles (i.e. DR4 subtypes) were identified, and only certain alleles (DRB1*0401, *0404, *0405, *0408) were associated with RA.[6,7] Thirdly, population studies revealed that RA was associated with DRB1 alleles other than DR4 subtypes (Table 1.1).

The RA shared epitope hypothesis – out of chaos comes order!

The plethora of HLA associations with RA argued strongly against DR4 as the sole explanation for RA and suggested that either multiple DRB1 alleles were RA DS genes or that these alleles were all in linkage disequilibrium with a single DS gene; both seemed unlikely. However, this was apparently resolved by the observation that RA-associated DRB1 alleles all contained a conserved sequence of amino acids (QKRAA/QRRAA/RRRAA) in their third hypervariable region[8–20] (Table 1.2).

In contrast, DR4 subtypes not associated with RA (DRB1*0402, *0403) do not contain these amino acid residues.[7] Considerable debate has occurred as to whether a valine or a glycine residue at amino acid position 86 is also important.[21] The association of this sequence with RA is now referred to as the 'RA shared epitope' (SE) hypothesis.[20] In Caucasoid populations the SE is observed in over 90% of RA patients, although it is also present in approximately half of the unaffected population.[7,22] Several suggestions have been put forward for the mechanism by which the SE determines RA susceptibility; these are based largely on the fact that the SE is in a part of the DR molecule that influences peptide presentation to the T-cell receptor (TCR) on CD4+ lymphocytes. The SE may:

- determine high-affinity binding of arthritogenic peptides;
- model the TCR repertoire towards a predisposition for generating an arthritogenic response;
- act as a receptor for an arthritogenic pathogen; or
- provide a site for antigenic cross reactivity with prokaryotic peptide sequences.

Although there is as yet no definitive proof for the SE in RA, the concept has now been widely accepted and, after almost 10 years, has entered into immunological dogma. The purpose of this review is to examine critically whether this hypothesis can accommodate epidemiological and immunogenetic findings relating to RA susceptibility and severity.

Table 1.2 Third hypervariable region sequences of HLA-DRB1 alleles associated with rheumatoid arthritis

DRB1	Amino acid sequence
*0101	QRRAA
*0102	QRRAA
*0401	QKRAA
*0404	QRRAA
*0405	QRRAA
*0408	QRRAA
*1402	QRRAA
*1001	RRRAA

Does RA prevalence correlate with 'baseline' frequencies of the SE in different populations?

RA has been described in most populations around the world[23] with a remarkably similar prevalence of approximately 1%, although there is evidence for some differences in prevalence between rural and urban cohorts of the same population.[24,25] Populations have also been described in which there is either a high prevalence of RA, e.g. some native North American populations,[26] or a low prevalence, e.g. Nigerian Africans[27] and Hong Kong Chinese.[28]

The frequency of HLA-DR4 and other DRB1 alleles carrying the SE sequence can vary dramatically between populations. In the UK, the frequency of the SE is high (approximately half the population) and this may in part explain the 1% RA prevalence observed. In Yakima and Tlingit North American Indians the reported high prevalence of RA correlates with the high frequency of the SE-positive allele DRB1*1402 in these populations (60% and 80%, respectively).[10,29] In contrast, in Nigerians, in whom RA is rare and, when diagnosed, usually follows a mild course,[30,31] we have determined that the SE is present in only 14% of the population.[27] This may provide an explanation for the observed epidemiology.

A relationship therefore appears to exist between SE frequency in the population and RA prevalence. This, together with the high correlation observed between different SE-bearing DRB1 alleles in a wide range of populations, provides as yet the strongest argument for the hypothesis that the SE encodes the RA risk.

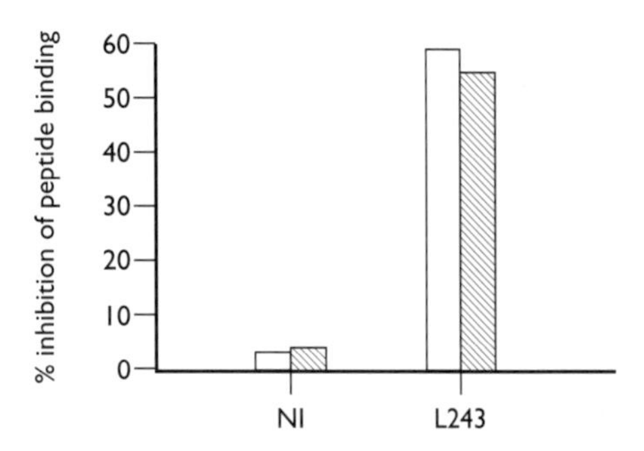

Figure 1.1 Inhibition of the binding of peptide HA 307–319 to SAVC (DRB1*0401; open bars) and DAL (DRB1*0402; hatched bars) Epstein–Barr virus cell lines with NI and L243 monoclonal antibodies.

Is there evidence for the QK/QRRAA sequence as an epitope recognized by the immune system?

The 'SE' is a linear sequence of amino acids and, as proteins form a tertiary structure, it is possible that only three-dimensional epitopes would be recognized and be functionally relevant. This does not appear to be the case for the QKRAA/QRRAA sequence and several monoclonal antibodies have been produced with reaction patterns determined by this sequence.[32,33] Furthermore, T-cell clones have been generated with reactivity restricted by residues within the SE.[34–36] These reports would suggest that the SE is a discrete entity that can be recognized immunogenetically.

Does the SE have more relevance in determination of peptide binding than interaction with the TCR?

As yet there is no evidence for an arthritogenic or joint-specific peptide in RA; the majority of peptides eluted from DR4 originate from either MHC molecules themselves or from other endogenous and ubiquitous self-proteins. In vitro experiments of peptide binding to HLA-DR suggest that a single immunogenetic peptide can bind to different HLA-DR molecules.[37] In addition, the crystal structure of the HLA-DR1–influenza peptide complex revealed that the backbone of DR1 binding stems from the conserved region of the molecule.[38] As the RA SE resides in a hypervariable region of the molecule, this would suggest that this sequence may be less important for peptide binding.

Our data obtained by fluorescence-activated cell sorter (FACS) analysis to measure the influence of the SE sequence in determination of peptide binding suggested that it had little or no effect (Figure 1.1). The binding of a biotinylated influenza peptide, HA 307–319 (PKYVKQNTLKLAT), a known T-cell epitope with an ability to bind a wide range of HLA-DR molecules,[34] was measured with the use of an SE-positive HLA-DRB1*0401 homozygous cell line (SAVC). Binding was not inhibited by preincubation with a monoclonal antibody (NI) recognizing the SE. In contrast, incubation with a pan-HLA-DR monoclonal antibody (L243) inhibited peptide binding. Exactly the same patterns of peptide binding and effects of monoclonal antibodies were observed for an SE-negative HLA-DRB1*0402 homozygous cell line (DAL). Experiments performed elsewhere with T-cell clones restricted by the SE region demonstrated that the same SE monoclonal antibody inhibited T-cell recognition. These results bring into question the role of the SE in the selective binding of an arthritogenic peptide, and they support studies that demonstrate the importance of the SE in interactions between HLA-DR molecules and the TCR.[34–36]

Alteration of the two amino acids at positions 70 (Q) and 71 (K) of a DRB1*0401 molecule remove HLA-restricted peptide recognition by specific T-cells.[34] If the SE is functionally important, it is likely to be concerned more with T-cell recognition than peptide binding. This is in keeping with other studies that have demonstrated that HLA-DR alleles are important in determining the T-cell receptor repertoire.[39] If this is the case, it would suggest that the search for clonal expansions of TCRs in RA is best restricted to patients with a well defined and homogeneous DR profile.

How does the evidence for molecular mimicry fit with the SE concept?

Sequence homology has been discovered between the QKRAA HV3 motif of DRB1*0401 and sequences from Epstein–Barr virus gp110, dnaJ heat-shock protein from *Escherichia coli*, and from several other bacteria.[40–42] RA patients have raised humoral and cellular responses to bacterial proteins containing this sequence, and this has suggested that 'multi-step molecular mimicry' mechanisms may be operating in RA.[43] Within the thymus, T cells with low-affinity recognition for self-DR peptides are positively selected. If these peptides resemble bacteria-derived peptides, subsequent immunization with complex bacterial proteins containing the sequence may preferentially expand such T cells. This immune response could be sustained and targeted to diathrodial sites of mechanical stress by expression of human heat-shock proteins resembling *E. coli* dnaJ. Although human dnaJ homologues do not contain the QKRAA sequence, they have sequence homology and immunological cross reactivity with *E. coli* dnaJ. Epitope spreading may be sufficient to trigger a response. Thus, human dnaJ homologues may represent the final target of T lymphocytes that have been selected positively by self HLA-derived QKRAA peptide and that have been later triggered by exogenous antigens.

This explanation concentrates on the DRB1*0401 molecule, which carries the QKRAA motif; the other SE-bearing alleles carrying QRRAA or RRRAA should also be considered. Clearly, if the immune system has difficulty in discriminating between these three motifs, the mechanism could apply equally to all the SE-bearing alleles. However, as will be discussed later, this cannot explain why individuals with the DRB1*0401/*0404 genotype have an increased risk for severe RA compared with those who are homozygous for DRB1*0401/ *0401.

Is the SE compatible with what we know about HLA and RA severity?

Before the concept of the SE in RA was introduced, we and others had already come to the conclusion that HLA-DR4 was related more to disease severity or progression than to susceptibility per se.[44] This appeared to be particularly clear in the extent of erosions.[45,46] Further support came from the observation that severe extra-articular forms of RA, including Felty's syndrome[47] and major vasculitis,[48] were associated with exceptionally high DR4 frequency, particularly DRB1*0401 (Dw4). Homozygosity for DR4 also appeared to be related to disease severity.[49,50]

Following the concept of the SE it became clear that, although homozygosity for the SE was associated with a higher risk for severe disease, the relationship between severity and the different DRB1 alleles carrying the SE sequence was not identical. By taking non-SE homozygosity (SE–/SE–) as a point of reference it was observed that the risk for severe RA in DRB1*0401/*0404 heterozygotes was exceptionally high (odds ratio 50).[22,51] This has been confirmed by a number of studies and may also apply to male patients and those with onset at a younger age.[22] As both male and young individuals represent groups that are normally 'protected' from RA, they presumably have a higher threshold for disease onset and require a stronger genetic input. Clearly the *0401/*0404 genotype represents the highest risk for severe disease although it is premature to use this information to determine therapeutic or clinical practice. Many RA patients without this genotype develop severe disease, and whilst DRB1* 0401/*0404 status may have high specificity for severe disease, its sensitivity is low.[52]

If the SE is a single entity that determines risk, the question remains as to why such variations in risk exist for different SE-bearing alleles and genotypes. As yet, this remains incompatible with the SE concept. One possible explanation may be that only one of these alleles encodes susceptibility for RA whereas the other encodes severity. This could conceivably be explained by the latter being in linkage disequilibrium (preferential haplotypic association) with high production of tumour necrosis factor-α (TNF-α).

The gene for TNF-α is a good candidate in RA, for which there is convincing evidence in support of its inflammatory and erosive role within the synovial joint.[53,54] Polymorphisms exist in the promoter region of TNF and appears to correlate with the level of gene expression.[55] The TNF-α level is likely to be highly relevent to disease expression; an association has been reported of such polymorphism with cerebral malaria in Africans.[56] A relationship between HLA haplotypes and the level of in vitro TNF-α production exists;[57] DR3 and some DR4-bearing haplotypes appear to correlate with high TNF-α production. HLA-DR2 has also been correlated with lower TNF-α production, which may be of relevence and explain why DR2 is negatively associated with erosive RA.[45] Recently we have used highly polymorphic microsatellite markers in the TNF region to establish whether HLA-DRB1-bearing haplotypes with particular TNF microsatellite profiles exist in RA patients.[58] Two DR4-bearing haplotypes were identified in RA patients:

- DRB1*0401-TNFd4-TNFa6-TNFb5-HLA-B44; and
- DRB1*0401-TNFd5-TNFc2-TNFa2-TNFb1-HLA-B62.

Although no DRB1*0404 haplotype was identified with a particular TNF microsatellite profile, the TNF-α2 allele was found at increased frequency in *0404 patients but not in those with *0401.[58] The TNF-α2 allele has previously been associated with high TNF-α production,[57] although clearly more investigation is required to clarify any relationship with RA severity.

Are certain SE-containing alleles associated with RA susceptibility, and others with severity or progression?

As detailed above, the involvement of HLA in RA is now considered to be more concerned with severity or disease progression. This is supported by community-based studies of RA prevalence[59] and RA incidence[60] where no association with DR4 or the SE was found. These studies suggest (1) that HLA-DR4 or the SE are more associated with those patients with disease severity that warrants attendance at a hospital clinic, and (2) that the frequencies of DR4 or the SE in incident RA cases will gradually increase over time in patients with persistent disease. The effect of HLA in such situations may be heterogeneous, with some SE-bearing alleles associated primarily with susceptibility.

In a recent study[61] we have HLA-DRB1 typed a further cohort of incident RA cases recruited to the Norfolk Arthritis Register.[62] As reported in an earlier study,[60] the frequency of DR4 and the SE did not differ significantly between RA cases at entry and controls. A marginal increase for DR4 was observed when just rheumatoid factor (RF) positive cases were considered (41.2% vs 34.3%), and this increased further for RF-positive cases with persistent RA at 1 year (47.1%). When subtypes of DR4 were considered, no differences in DRB1*0401 frequency were observed for the above groups. Interestingly an increase in DRB1*0404 was apparent in cases with RA at entry vs controls (14.7% vs 4.4%). This was higher in RF-positive cases (23.5%) and rose further (29.4%) in RF-positive RA cases at 1 year. These data suggest that DRB1*0404 may be associated with onset or early disease, and that it is DRB1*0401 which gradually increases over time and is associated with progression. This interpretation is not compatible with the concept of a single SE in RA.

Is clinical heterogeneity in RA compatible with the SE hypothesis?

If the SE represents a homogeneous risk factor for RA, with no other HLA-encoded genes making a contribution to the disease process, one would predict that any clinical heterogeneity observed in RA would be due to non-HLA-encoded genes or environmental effects.

In RA, various clinical features appear to be predominantly associated with particular SE-containing alleles. RA patients with a long-term seronegative RF profile are associated with DR1 and not DR4.[63] The extra-articular manifestation of Felty's syndrome is predominantly with DRB1*0401[64] and is often found in haplotypic association with the complement C4 null allele C4B*QO,[65] HLA-B44, and TAP2D.[66] In both Greeks and Hong Kong Chinese[67] Felty's syndrome is a rare complication of RA and this may relate to the paucity of DRB1*0401 or particular DRB1*0401-bearing haplotypes in these populations. Such data suggest that in addition to the requirement of the SE (or perhaps even instead of it) other HLA region encoded genes are necessary for some features of disease expression.

Does genetic analysis indicate that the SE is acting as a single susceptibility gene in RA?

This question was considered recently and prompted a detailed genetic analysis of RA data.[67] Various models for the involvement of HLA in RA susceptibility were examined and two main hypotheses were considered, one assuming the involvement of HLA-DR alleles themselves and the other assuming the involvement of a linked locus. In the former, the direct involvement of the SE sequence was examined with the assumption that the effect of DR was due only to the presence of the SE and that all SE-bearing alleles had the same effect. The model for equality of association of a susceptibility allele and three HLA-DR alleles (*0401, *0404, *0101) was strongly rejected. Furthermore, the model for a two-epitope hypothesis (one epitope QKRAA for *0401 and a second QRRAA for *0404 and *0101) was also rejected.

In contrast, a model for susceptibility alleles in linkage disequilibrium with HLA-DR could not be rejected, and the coupling frequency (a measure of allelic association) was highest for DRB1*0404, less for *0401, and lowest for *0101. The conclusion was drawn that there was one RA susceptibility allele at a bi-allelic locus in linkage disequilibrium with DRB1*0404, *0401 and *0101. A dominant model was rejected, but the data were compatible with a recessive mode of inheritance, in line with a previous report.[68]

This approach to the analysis of the contribution of HLA in RA provides evidence clearly at odds with the accepted perception of how the SE is implicated in RA. If this evidence is correct, other explanations for what constitutes DS genes in RA are required.

Can other explanations be given for HLA associations with RA?

Recently a number of studies have suggested new lines of investigation for the role of HLA in RA susceptibility. Whilst these remain speculative, any data that force us critically to re-evaluate the role of the DRB1 SE in RA should be considered, and new hypotheses encouraged.

Genetic differences in HLA-encoded susceptibility between males and females suggest HLA-linked DS genes

A clear difference exists in RA susceptibility between males and females, with RA in the latter being at least twice as prevalent. This is usually attributed to an involvement of hormonal factors. What is not perhaps appreciated is that HLA associations with RA differ between males and females. A higher frequency of HLA-B62-DRB1*0401 haplotypes is observed in males[69] and HLA-B44-DRB1*0401 haplotypes in females. We have recently confirmed these observations in further cohorts and identified particular TNF microsatellite profiles for each haplotype.[70]

These observations can be explained in two ways: either (1) the HLA-B62-DRB1*0401 haplotype represents a high-risk RA haplotype and, as males are usually protected, a higher frequency would be expected in males who develop RA; or (2) the HLA-B62 haplotype contains genes specifically implicated in the development of RA in males. We have favoured the latter explanation, largely on the basis of the circumstantial evidence that:

- the level of testosterone in both men[71] and mice[72] is influenced by genes encoded within the MHC;
- HLA-B62 is associated with lower testosterone levels in both healthy males and those with RA;[73] and
- low testosterone levels exist in male RA patients, independently of treatment.[74]

The gene(s) responsible for such effects represents a good candidate as an RA DS gene in males.

In females, a similar situation could apply. Recent studies have confirmed a relationship between breast-feeding and increased risk for RA in females.[75] This together with other studies implicates a possible role for prolactin – an immunomodulatory hormone. The gene for prolactin maps at the telomeric boundary of the HLA region and data now suggest that linkage disequilibrium extends from class II HLA genes to the prolactin gene; this has been confirmed for an HLA-B44-DRB1*0401 haplotype (AH Hajeer et al, unpublished data). A polymorphism of the prolactin gene has already been identified,[76] and we have suggested recently that regulatory polymorphisms in the prolactin gene may be in linkage disequilibrium with particular HLA haplotypes.[77] This could explain the development of autoimmunity in females.

HLA-DRB1*0401 may directly influence antigen processing pathways relevant to RA

A recent study conducted by the group of Roudier[78] used synthetic peptides corresponding to the third hypervariable regions (HV3) of DRB1 molecules to prepare affinity columns to screen bacterial lysates of *E. coli*. They found that HV3 peptides containing QKRAA (DRB1*0401) and RRRAA (DRB1*1001) specifically bound the bacterial 70-kDa heat-shock protein dnaK. Further experiments revealed that the human constitutive 70-kDa heat-shock protein hsp73 co-precipitates only with DRB1*0401 and *1001; hsp73 appears to associate with immature complexes of the HLA-DR α/β heterodimer and invariant chain at an early stage of synthesis in the endoplasmic reticulum and this continues independently of the maturation process. Examination of lysosomal fractions revealed that hsp73 was also associated with DRB1*0401 and DRB1*1001 heterodimers lacking the invariant chain. This suggests that the association of hsp73 with DRB1*0401 and *1001 molecules may specifically affect their intracellular trafficking and the way in which they interact with peptide fragments. Such effects may:

- impair DR cell-surface expression;
- competitively inhibit the lysosomal transport of any proteins containing QKRAA or RRRAA motifs (for example Epstein–Barr virus gp110, which contains QKRAA);
- lead to hsp73 autoimmunization; and
- enhance proteolysis in lysosomes and allow HV3 peptides to be presented to the immune system, thus influencing thymic selection. This is possible, as it has previously been demonstrated that DRB1*0401-positive individuals are tolerant to the QKRAA peptide sequence.[79]

Clearly, the specific binding properties of hsp73 to DRB1*0401 and *1001 may be implicated in

RA aetiopathology through any of the mechanisms suggested above, and further work is required in this area.

Does the HLA association with RA reside with DQ or DR?

A recent review has suggested that RA susceptibility is really encoded by HLA-DQ alleles and that HLA-DRB1 operates as a protective locus.[80] These ideas have largely come from studies of collagen-induced arthritis in congenic and H2 recombinant mice. Mice lacking a functional H-2E molecule (DRB1 equivalent) are susceptible to collagen-induced arthritis, due to the presence of a predisposing H-2A molecule (DQ equivalent). Offspring of these mice mated with a range of H2 transgenic mice carrying various E beta genes revealed that the Eb^d allele (amino acids D and A at positions 70 and 71, respectively) conferred protection, whilst others did not.

Although collagen-induced arthritis is a poor animal model for RA aetiology, these results may point towards a mechanism operating in human disease. Zanelli and colleagues[80] have suggested that protection by some DR molecules is dominant over DQ-mediated susceptibility and that in most cases the disease will progress only if the non-protective DRB1 specificity is carried on both chromosomes. The proposed mechanism by which DRB1 molecules protect is through provision of a source of DRB1 peptides presented by DQ molecules. In support of this concept Zanelli used double-transgenic DQB1*0302/DQA1*0301 mice and found that they could present protective HV3 peptides of DRB1*1501 (DR2) and DRB1*0402 (Dw10) but not the non-protective HV3 peptides from DRB1*0101 and DRB1*0401. These experiments raise some interesting issues, but do not fit completely with all population associations of HLA and RA. For example, RA in the Japanese is associated primarily with DRB1*0405 (Dw15), which is in strong linkage disequilibrium with the DQw4 molecule.[81]

CONCLUSION

The SE hypothesis is based on the firm foundation that it is a functionally and immunologically relevant motif. Furthermore, it accommodates most of the HLA/RA associations observed in different populations, and it is understandable that this concept has gained such support over the last nine years.

In contrast, genetic analysis rejects this hypothesis, and it cannot accommodate many of the observations regarding HLA and RA severity and clinical heterogeneity. It is important to maintain a level of scepticism regarding the SE and to consider new ways in which the HLA complex may contribute to RA susceptibility and disease expression. Great effort is now being made to identify non-HLA DS genes in RA and it is possible that HLA, the first DS to be found for RA, may be the last to be fully understood.

REFERENCES

1. Silman AJ, MacGregor A, Thomson W, Holligan S, Carthy D, Ollier WER. Twin concordance rates for rheumatoid arthritis: results of a nation-wide study. *Br J Rheumatol* 1993; **32**:903–7.
2. Aho K, Markku K, Tuominen J, Kaprio J. Occurrence of rheumatoid arthritis in a nationwide series of twins. *J Rheumatol* 1986; **13**:899–902.
3. Winchester RJ. B-lymphocyte allo-antigens, cellular expression and disease significance with special reference to rheumatoid arthritis. *Arthritis Rheum* 1977; **20**:159.
4. Stastny P. Association of B-cell alloantigen DRw4 with rheumatoid arthritis. *N Engl J Med* 1978; **298**:869–71.
5. Deighton CM, Walker DJ, Griffiths ID, Roberts DF. The contribution of HLA to rheumatoid arthritis. *Clin Genet* 1989; **36**:178–82.
6. Ollier W, Carthy D, Cutbush S et al. HLA-DR4 associated Dw types in rheumatoid arthritis. *Tissue Antigens* 1988; **33**:30–7.

7. Ollier W, Thomson W. Population genetics of rheumatoid arthritis. *Rheum Dis Clin North Am* 1992; **18**:741–59.
8. Ollier WER, Stephens C, Awad J et al. Is rheumatoid arthritis in Indians associated with HLA antigens sharing a DRβ1 epitope? *Ann Rheum Dis* 1991; **50**:295–7.
9. Nichol FE, Woodrow J. HLA-DR antigens in Indian patients with rheumatoid arthritis. *Lancet* 1981; **i**:220–1.
10. Wilkens RF, Nepom GT, Marks CR et al. Associations of HLA-Dw16 with rheumatoid arthritis in Yakima Indians. *Arthritis Rheum* 1991; **34**:43–7.
11. Choremi H, Iniotaki A, Piskontaki I, Sfikakis P. Association of HLA-DR1 in Greek rheumatoid arthritis patients. In: *Proceedings of the 11th International Histocompatibility Workshop and Conference, Yokahama, 1991*; Oxford University Press: Oxford, 1992 PS-12-3:176.
12. Carthy D, Ollier W, Papasteriades C, Pappas H, Thomson W. A shared HLA-DRB1 sequence confers RA susceptibility in Greeks. *Eur J Immunogenet* 1993; **20**:391–8.
13. Nunez-Roldan A, Arguer-Zuazua E, Villechonous-pineda E, de la Prada-Arroyo M. Estudious de los antigenous HLA-DR en la arthritis reumatoidea. *Rev Esp Rheum* 1982; **9**:9–11.
14. Sanchez B, Moreno I, Magarino R et al. HLA-DRw10 confers the highest susceptibility to rheumatoid arthritis in a Spanish population. *Tissue Antigens* 1990; **36**:174–6.
15. De Juan MD, Belmonte I, Barado J et al. Differential associations of HLA-DR antigens with rheumatoid arthritis (RA) in Basques: High frequency of DR1 and DR10 and lack of association with HLA-DR4 or any of its subtypes. *Tissue Antigens* 1994; **43**:320–3.
16. Stastny P. Joint report on rheumatoid arthritis. In: *Histocompatibility Testing* (Terasaki PI, ed.). UCLA Tissue Typing Laboratory: Los Angeles, 1980:681–6.
17. Gao X, Gazit E, Lirnch A, Stastny P. Rheumatoid arthritis in Israeli Jews; association with two sequences shared by several DRB1 alleles in the third hypervariable region. [abstract]. *Hum Immunol* 1990; **29**:69.
18. Cutbush SD, Chikanza IC, Lutalo S et al. Sequence-specific oligonucleotide typing in Shona patients with rheumatoid arthritis and healthy controls from Zimbabwe. *Tissue Antigens* 1993; **41**:169–72.
19. Pile KD, Tikly M, Bell JI, Wordsworth BP. HLA-DR antigens and rheumatoid arthritis in black South Africans: A study of ethnic groups. *Tissue Antigens* 1992; **39**:138–40.
20. Gregersen PK, Silver J, Winchester RJ. The shared epitope hypothesis: an approach to understanding the molecular genetics of susceptibility to rheumatoid arthritis. *Arthritis Rheum* 1987; **30**:1205–1213.
21. Nelson JL, Mickelson EM, Masewicz SA et al. Dw14 (DRB1*0404) is a Dw4-dependent risk factor for rheumatoid arthritis. *Tissue Antigens* 1991; **38**:145–51.
22. MacGregor A, Ollier W, Thomson W, Jawaheer D, Silman AJ. HLA-DRB1*0401/0404 genotype and rheumatoid arthritis: increased association in men, young age at onset, and disease severity. *J Rheumatol* 1995; **22**:1032–6.
23. Silman AJ, Hochberg MC. *Epidemiology of the Rheumatic Diseases*. Oxford University Press: Oxford, 1993.
24. Bighton SW, de la Harpe AL, van Staden DJ, Badenhorst JH, Meyers OL. The prevalence of rheumatoid arthritis in a rural African population. *J Rheumatol* 1988; **15**:405–8.
25. Solomon L, Robin G, Valkenburg HA. Rheumatoid arthritis in an urban South African Negro population. *Ann Rheum Dis* 1975; **34**:128–35.
26. Harvey J, Lotze M, Stevens MB, Lambert G, Jacobson D. Rheumatoid arthritis in a Chippewa band. I. Pilot screening study of disease prevalence. *Arthritis Rheum* 1981; **24**:717–21.
27. Silman AJ, Ollier WER, Adebajo A et al. Absence of rheumatoid arthritis in a rural Nigerian population. *J Rheumatol* 1993; **20**:618–22.
28. Lau E, Symmons D, Bankhead C, MacGregor A, Donnan S, Silman A. Low prevalence of rheumatoid arthritis in the urbanized Chinese of Hong Kong. *J Rheumatol* 1993; **20**:1133–7.
29. Nelson JL, Boyer GS, Templin DW et al, Rheumatoid arthritis and HLA antigens in Tlingit Indians. In: *Proceedings of the 11th International Histocompatibility Workshop and Conference, Yokahama, 1991*; Oxford University Press: Oxford 1992 PS-12-12:180.
30. Greenwood BM. Polyarthritis in Western Nigeria. I. Rheumatoid arthritis. *Ann Rheum Dis* 1969; **28**:488–96.
31. Greenwood BM. Low incidence of rheumatoid factor and autoantibodies in Nigeria patients with rheumatoid arthritis. *Br Med J* 1970; **1**:71–3.
32. Lee SH, Gregersen PK, Shen HH et al. Strong

association of rheumatoid arthritis with the presence of a polymorphic Ia epitope defined by a monoclonal antibody; comparison with the derterminant DR4. *Rheumatol Int* 1984; **4**:17–23.
33. Yendle JE, Bowerman PD, Yousaf K et al. Production of a cytotoxic human monoclonal antibody with specificity for HLA-DR4 and DRw 10 by cells derived from a highly sensitized kidney recipient. *Hum Immunol* 1990; **27**:167–81.
34. Barber LD, Bal V, Lamb JR et al. Contribution of T-cell receptor-contacting and peptide-binding residues of the class II molecule HLA-DR4 Dw 10 to serologic and antigen-specific T-cell recognition. *Hum Immunol* 1992; **32**:110–18.
35. Tuosto L, Karr RW, Fu XT et al. Different regions of the *N*-terminal domains of HLA-DR1 influence recognition of individual peptide-DR1 complexes. *Hum Immunol* 1994; **40**:312–22.
36. Fu XT, Bono CP, Woulfe SL et al. Pocket of the HLA-DR (alpha,beta-1-*0401) molecule is a major determinant of T-cell recognition of peptide. *J Exp Med* 1995; **181**:915–26.
37. Busch R, Strang G, Howland K et al. Degenerate binding of immunogenic peptides to HLA-DR proteins on B cell surfaces. *Intern Immunol* 1990; **5**:443–51.
38. Stein LJ, Brown JH, Jardetzky TS et al. Crystal structure of the human class II MHC protein HLA-DR1 complexed with influenza virus peptide. *Nature* 1994; **386**:215–21.
39. Bhayani HE, Hedrick SM. The role of polymorphic amino acids of the MHC molecules in the selection of the T-cell repertoire. *J Immunol* 1991; **146**:1093–8.
40. Roudier J, Petersen J, Rhodes G et al. Susceptibility to rheumatoid arthritis maps to a T-cell epitope shared by the HLA Dw4 DR beta 1 chain and the Epstein–Barr virus glyco-protein gp110. *Proc Natl Acad Sci USA* 1989; **86**:5104–8.
41. Roudier J, Rhodes G, Petersen J et al. The Epstein–Barr virus glycoprotein gp110 a molecular link between HLA-DR4, HLA-DR1 and rheumatoid arthritis. *Scand J Immunol* 1988; **27**:367–71.
42. Albani S, Tuckwell JE, Esparza L et al. The susceptibility to rheumatoid arthritis is a cross-reactive B cell epitope shared by the *Escherichia coli* heat shock protein dnaJ and the histocompatibility leukocyte antigen DRB1*0401 molecule. *J Clin Invest* 1992; **89**:327–31.
43. Albani S, Keystone EC, Nelson JL et al. Positive selection in autoimmunity: Abnormal immune responses to a bacterial dnaJ antigenic determinant in patients with early rheumatoid arthritis. *Nature Med* 1995; **1**:448–52.
44. Jaraquemada D, Ollier W, Awad J, Young A, Festenstein H. HLA and rheumatoid arthritis: susceptibility or severity? *Dis Markers* 1986; **4**:43–53.
45. Young A, Jaraquemada D, Awad J et al. Association of the HLA-DR4/Dw4 and DR2/Dw2 with radiological changes in a prospective study of patients with rheumatoid arthritis. *Arthritis Rheum* 1984; **26**:511.
46. Jaraquemada D, Ollier W, Awad J et al. HLA and rheumatoid arthritis: a combined analysis of 440 British patients. *Ann Rheum Dis* 1989; **45**:627–36.
47. Klouda PT, Corbin SA, Bidwell JL et al. Felty's syndrome and HLA-DR antigens. *Tissue Antigens* 1986; **27**:112–3.
48. Scott DGI, Bacon PA, Tribe CR. Systemic rheumatoid vasculitis: A clinical and laboratory study of 50 cases. *Medicine* 1981; **60**:288–97.
49. Weyand CM, Hicok KC, Conn DL, Goronzy JJ. The influence of HLA-DRB1 genes on disease severity in rheumatoid arthritis. *Ann Intern Med* 1992; **117**:801–6.
50. Weyand CM, Xie CP, Goronzy JJ. Homozygosity for the HLA-DRB1 allele selected for extra articular manifestations in rheumatoid arthritis. *J Clin Invest* 1992; **89**:2033–9.
51. Wordsworth P, Pile KD, Buckely JD et al. HLA heterozygosity contributes to susceptibility to rheumatoid arthritis. *Am J Hum Genet* 1992; **51**:585–91.
52. Symmons D, Ollier WER, Brennan P, Silman AJ. Should patients with recent onset rheumatoid arthritis be offered genetic screening? *Ann Rheum Dis* 1996; **55**:407–10.
53. Brennan FM, Field M, Chu CQ, Feldmann M, Maini RN. Cytokine expression in rheumatoid arthritis. *Br J Rheumatol* 1991; **30**:76–80.
54. Elliott MJ, Maini RN, Feldmann M et al. Repeated therapy with monoclonal antibody to tumour necrosis factor a (cA2) in patients with rheumatoid arthritis. *Lancet* 1994; **344**:1125–7.
55. Wilson AG, Symons JA, McDowell TL, Di Giovine FS, Duff GW. Effects of a tumour necrosis factor (TNFα) promoter base transition on transcriptional activity. *Br J Rheum* 1994; **33**:89.
56. McGuire W, Hill AVS, Allsopp CEM, Greenwood BM, Kwiatkowski D. Variations in the TNF promoter region associated with

susceptibility to cerebral malaria. *Nature* 1994; **371**:508–11.

57. Pociot F, Briant L, Jongeneel CV et al. Association of tumor necrosis factor (TNF) and class II major histocompatibility complex alleles with the secretion of TNF-α and TNF-β by human mononuclear cells: a possible link to insulin dependent diabetes mellitus. *Eur J Immunol* 1993; **23**:224–31.
58. Hajeer A, Worthington J, Silman AJ, Ollier WER. TNF microsatellite polymorphisms are associated with HLA-DRB1*04 bearing haplotypes in RA patients. *Arthritis Rheum* 1996; **39**:1109–14.
59. DeJongh BM, van Romunde KJ, Valkenberg HA et al. Epidemiological study of HLA and GM in rheumatoid arthritis and related symptoms in an open Dutch population. *Ann Rheum Dis* 1984; **43**:613–19.
60. Thomson W, Pepper L, Payton A et al. Absence of an association between HLA-DRB1*04 and RA in newly diagnosed cases from the community. *Ann Rheum Dis* 1993; **52**:539–41.
61. Jawaheer D. Genetically encoded susceptibility to rheumatoid arthritis. PhD Thesis, University of Manchester, 1995.
62. Symmons DPM, Barrett EM, Scott DGI, Silman AJ. The Norfolk arthritis register – study of the incidence of RA. *Br J Rheumatol* 1990; **29**:79.
63. Stastny P, Olsen N, Pincus T et al. DR4 and DR1 define different subsets of patients with rheumatoid arthritis. In: *Immunology of HLA II* (Dupont B, ed.). Springer-Verlag: New York, 1989:418–19.
64. Hillarby MC, Hopkins J, Grennan DM. A reanalysis of the association between rheumatoid arthritis and without extra-articular features, HLA-DR4 and DR4 subtypes. *Tissue Antigens* 1991; **37**:39–41.
65. Hillarby MC, Clarkson R, Grennan DM et al. Immunogenetic heterogeneity in rheumatoid disease as illustrated by different MHC associations (DQ, Dw and C4) in articular and extra-articular subsets. *Br J Rheumatol* 1991; **30**:5–9.
66. Hillarby MC, Davies EJ, Donn RP, Grennan DM, Ollier WER, TAP2D is associated with HLA-B44 and DR4 and may contribute to rheumatoid arthritis and Felty's syndrome susceptibility. *Clin Exp Rheumatol* 1996; **14**:67–70.
67. Dizier MH, Eliaou JF, Babron MC, Combe B, Sany J, Clot J, Clerget-Dapoux F. Investigation of the HLA component involved in rheumatoid arthritis (RA) by using the marker association-segregation X^2 (MASC) method: Rejection of the unifying-shared-epitope hypothesis. *Am J Hum Genet* 1993; **53**:715–21.
68. Rigby AS, Silman AJ, Voelm L et al. Investigating the HLA component in rheumatoid arthritis an additive (dominant) mode of inheritance is rejected, a recessive mode is preferred. *Genet Epidemiol* 1991; **8**:153–75.
69. Ollier W, Venables PJW, Mumford PA et al. HLA antigen association with extra articular rheumatoid arthritis. *Tissue Antigens* 1984; **24**:279–91.
70. Hajeer A, John S, Ollier W et al. TNF microsatellite haplotypes are different in male and female RA patients. *J Rheumatol*. In press.
71. Spector TD, Ollier WER, Perry LA, Silman AJ. Evidence for similarity in testosterone levels in haplotype identical brothers. *Dis Markers* 1988; **6**:119–25.
72. Ivanyi P, Hampl R, Starka L, Mickova M, Genetic association between H-2 gene and testosterone metabolism in mice. *Nature New Biol* 1972; **238**:280–1.
73. Ollier W, Spector T, Silman A et al. Are certain HLA haplotypes responsible for low testosterone levels in males? *Dis Markers* 1989; **7**: 139–43.
74. Spector TD, Perry LA, Tubb G, Silman AJ, Huskisson EC. Low free testosterone levels in males with rheumatoid arthritis. *Ann Rheum Dis* 1988; **47**:65–8.
75. Brennan P, Silman A. Breast feeding and the onset of rheumatoid arthritis. *Arthritis Rheum* 1994; **37**:808–13.
76. Myal Y, DiMattia GE, Gregory CA, Friesen HG, Hamerton JL, Shiu RPC. A BglI RFLP at the human prolactin gene locus on chromosome 6. *Nucleic Acids Res* 1991; **19**:1167.
77. Brennan P, Ollier B, Worthington J, Hajeer A, Silman A. Are both genetic and reproductive association with rheumatoid arthritis linked to prolactin? *Lancet* 1996; **348**:106–9.
78. Auger I, Escola JM, Gorval JP, Roudier J. HLA-DR4 and HLA-DR10 motifs that carry susceptibility to rheumatoid arthritis bind 70-kD heat shock proteins. *Nature Med* 1996; **2**:306–10.
79. Salvat S, Auger I, Rochelle L et al. Tolerance to a self peptide from the third hypervariable region of HLA-DRB1*0401 in rheumatoid arthritis patients and normal subjects. *J Immunol* 1994; **153**:5321–9.
80. Zanelli, E, Gonzalez-Gay MA, David CS. Could HLA-DRB1 be the protective locus in rheumatoid arthritis? *Immunol Today* 1995; **16**:274–8.

81. Otha N, Nishimura IK, Tanimoto K et al. Association between HLA and Japanese patients with rheumatoid arthritis. *Hum Immunol* 1982; **5**:123–32.

2

Heat-shock proteins and arthritis – has the hot air now subsided?

Thomas Kamradt, Andreas Krause, Gerd-R Burmester

INTRODUCTION

Infectious agents are regarded as major environmental factors able to cause chronic inflammatory arthritides. An infectious trigger is established clearly for some arthritides, e.g. viral arthritides, rheumatic fever, the reactive arthritides, Lyme borreliosis, arthritis associated with HIV infection, tuberculosis or leprosy, and arthritis in Whipple's disease. In addition, arthritis sometimes occurs after immunization; and infections, such as HIV, can drastically influence the clinical course of pre-existing inflammatory arthritis. Finally, it has long been speculated that rheumatoid arthritis might be triggered by an infectious agent.[1] If infections trigger chronic inflammatory arthritis, two hypotheses, which are not mutually exclusive, need to be considered: persistent infection and infection-induced immunopathology.[2,3] One possible mechanism of infection-induced immunopathology is molecular mimicry: this hypothesis suggests that potentially self-reactive lymphocytes which are normally tolerant become activated by microbial antigens sharing some degree of sequence homology with a self-antigen. Once activated, these lymphocytes continue to cause tissue damage, either directly or via activation of accessory cells.[4–7] Heat-shock proteins (hsp), with their high degree of homology between eukaryotes and prokaryotes seemed natural suspects for the induction of molecular mimicry. The appearance of numerous reports on the immunological cross reactivity between mycobacterial and mammalian hsp60[8–12] led to the hypothesis that autoimmunity might be induced by cross reactive T cells recognizing both bacterial and host hsp. Here, we review the current evidence for and against a role for hsp in the pathogenesis of arthritides.

HEAT-SHOCK PROTEINS

Heat-shock proteins consist of a family of more than 25 members, ranging in molecular weight from 15 to 110 kDa. They are grouped according to their molecular weight to comprise an hsp60 family, an hsp70 family, etc. Members of each group often share similar functions and display high degrees of sequence homology.[13,14] Hsp are expressed in almost all eukaryotic and prokaryotic cells, both constitutively and inducibly. Hsp show a high degree of sequence homology between species as distantly related as bacteria and humans.[15] They were discovered over 30 years ago, when it was found that raising the temperature of the fruitfly *Drosophila melanogaster* above a certain level induced the enhanced expression of some genes. The proteins encoded by these genes were appropriately named 'heat-shock proteins'. A more accurate but less commonly used term is 'stress proteins', since hsp can be induced by a variety of stimuli in vitro and in vivo, including metabolic poisons, free radicals, cytokines, infection, ischaemia, and reperfusion.[16] All these insults potentially result in the accumulation of improperly folded proteins. Hsp help to remove or restructure these proteins.[17]

Hsp are expressed constitutively in normal cells, where they work as 'chaperonins', facilitating protein folding and intracellular transport,[18,19] including processing of peptide antigens for presentation to T cells.[20] Genes encoding two members of the hsp70 family are located within the major histocompatibility complex (MHC) region[21] and the MHC class I peptide-binding cleft shows a high degree of homology to the corresponding sequence of hsp70.[22] Furthermore, hsp70 chaperones proteins into lysosomes.[23] More recently it was shown that members of the hsp90 family can chaperone exogenous antigens into the endogenous pathway of antigen presentation by MHC class I molecules, thus leading to recognition of these antigens by CD8+ T lymphocytes.[24,25] This is an important finding, since the default pathway for exogenous antigens is presentation by MHC class II molecules and recognition by CD4+ T lymphocytes. Finally, hsp are essential components of several signal transduction pathways,[26] and host hsp are sometimes exploited by pathogens for their own replication.[27]

In some bacteria the production of hsp is upregulated upon infection of macrophages[28] and microbial hsp elicit strong immune responses in a variety of infections (reviewed in references 13 and 14). Yet, surprisingly in view of this strong immunogenicity, microbial hsp are highly homologous to human hsp. The hsp60 families of humans and *Mycobacterium tuberculosis*, for example, share 48% sequence identity, with conservative amino acid exchanges accounting for a significant proportion of the nonidentical sequence stretches.[29] It is this high degree of conservation that has made hsp so attractive for immunologists and probably also for the immune system itself. The hsp of any vertebrate host will be homologous to hsp of invading microorganisms and to the hsp of ingested plants or animals (food). From an immunological viewpoint, therefore, hsp are at the crossroads of self and nonself. This is interesting not only for immunologists probing the realms of 'tolerance, danger, and the extended family'[30] but also for any organism trying to defend itself against invaders while avoiding the *horror autotoxicus*. It seems that the immune system is confronted with the dilemma of either restricting the immune response to self-hsp so strictly that it might not be able to recognize some pathogen's hsp, or recognizing foreign hsp so avidly that the spectre of autoimmunity arises. It is this problem that has generated so much interest and research activity on hsp.

The immune response to hsp has been invoked in the pathogenesis of a variety of autoimmune diseases, chronic sequelae of infectious diseases (reviewed in references 9, 13, 14, 31 and 32), and even atherosclerosis.[33] Here, we will focus on recent findings regarding the potential role – pathogenic or protective – of hsp65 in arthritides. Nevertheless, two other hsp have been linked to rheumatic diseases, namely hsp90 with systemic lupus erythematodes[34] and hsp73 with mixed connective tissue disease.[35]

ADJUVANT ARTHRITIS IN RATS

The first evidence for an involvement of hsp in arthritis came from an animal model, adjuvant arthritis (AA). AA can be induced in susceptible strains of rats by immunization with a mixture of mineral oil and mycobacteria.[36] T-cell lines that transfer the disease to naive syngeneic recipients can be derived from diseased rats.[37] Analysis of one such rat T-cell line, A2b, revealed that it recognized amino acid residues 180–188 on mycobacterial hsp65 and a cross reactive antigen on cartilage proteoglycan.[38,39] The logical next step was trying to induce AA by immunization with mycobacterial hsp65 in mineral oil to test the hypothesis that T-cell reactivity against hsp65 was responsible for the induction of arthritis. However, it was found that immunization with hsp65 did not induce arthritis but instead protected rats from subsequent attempts at arthritis induction with complete Freund's adjuvant.[39,40] Furthermore, adoptive transfer of spleen cells from hsp65-immunized rats into naive syngeneic recipients provided protection against AA.[41] Vaccination with the 180–188 peptide itself protected rats against AA in some studies[42] but not others.[43] Likewise, infection with recombinant vaccinia viruses expressing either mycobacterial hsp65[44] or human hsp60[45,46] also protected rats from AA. The latter finding is important, since the 180–188 epitope of mycobacterial hsp65 is not conserved, i.e., this sequence is not found on the human hsp60.[29]

Immunization with hsp65 protected rats not only against adjuvant arthritis, but also against some forms of experimentally induced arthritis in which mycobacterial antigens are not thought to play a role; this includes arthritis induced by streptococcal cell walls,[47] or type II collagen.[40] Hsp65 immunization also protected mice against pristane-induced arthritis.[48] Similar protective effects have recently been described for the mycobacterial hsp70[49] and hsp10.[50] Even more striking was the demonstration that *Yersinia*-associated arthritis in rats could be suppressed not only by immunization with mycobacterial hsp65 in mineral oil but also by bovine serum albumin or saline given in mineral oil.[51] In the light of these results it is difficult to imagine a direct role for mycobacterial hsp65 in the pathogenesis of experimental arthritis in rats. How could a ubiquitous hsp be responsible for organ-specific autoimmune diseases? What is the role for organ-specific antigens? Further undermining the concept of a direct role for hsp65 in the pathogenesis of arthritis was the finding that immunological tolerance of type II collagen could prevent AA in rats.[52] Although it is not clear what role, if any, type II collagen plays in the pathogenesis of arthritis, pathogenetically important organ-specific autoantigens have been defined in other autoimmune diseases. Insulin-dependent diabetes mellitus (IDDM) in NOD mice can be influenced dramatically by injection of mycobacterial, murine or human hsp.[31,53,54] Nevertheless, at least one autoantigen which definitely plays an important role in the induction of IDDM has been identified,[55,56] and similar findings are to be expected for autoimmune arthritis. What, then, is the effect of immunity to hsp in adjuvant arthritis?

Recently, van Eden and colleagues have examined the mechanisms by which hsp65 immunization protects rats against AA. They identified eight synthetic peptides derived from mycobacterial hsp65 which elicited T-cell responses in Lewis rats.[57] Of these, only the peptide corresponding to mycobacterial hsp65 amino acid residues 256–270 induced protection against AA. Adoptive transfer of a T-cell line specific for the 256–270 peptide also mediated protection. Most importantly, the 256–270 peptide activated T cells which also recognized the homologous 256–270 sequence of rat hsp60. Furthermore, these T cells also responded to heat-shocked syngeneic antigen-presenting cells (APC). Importantly, immunization with the rat 256–270 peptide did not confer protection. Fine specificity analysis of T-cell lines derived after immunization with either mycobacterial or rat hsp peptide 256–270 revealed that T cells primed with the mycobacterial 256–270 peptide recognized the cross reactive 256–265 core epitope, whereas immunization with the rat 256–270 peptide-primed T cells recognized the rat-specific 261–270 core epitope[43] (see Figure 2.1).

This finding is important in that it demonstrates a protective rather than a pathogenic effect of self-reactive, i.e. autoimmune, T cells. Furthermore, it shows that bacterial hsp can induce T cells that are cross reactive with self-hsp. The observed cross reactivity with self-hsp60 offers an explanation for the earlier findings which demonstrated that preimmunization with mycobacterial hsp65 protected rodents against arthritis that was not induced by mycobacteria.[40,47,48] Since hsp60 expression is upregulated in arthritic joints in rats,[58,59] and self-hsp60-specific T cells can be activated by a variety of inflammatory stimuli,[12] it might be expected that T cells recognizing this antigen would downregulate inflammatory responses. In support of this interpretation is the earlier finding that vaccination with a peptide corresponding to mouse hsp60 amino acid residues

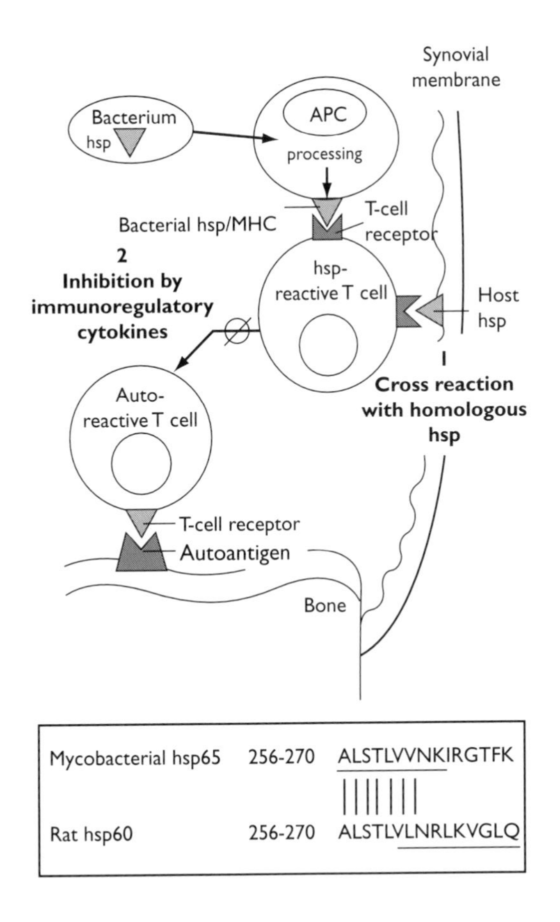

Figure 2.1 Hypotheses for the role of heat-shock proteins (hsp) in arthritis. The high degree of sequence homologies between bacterial and mammalian hsp led to the hypothesis of infection-induced autoimmunity by cross reactive T cells (see text). However, the adjuvant arthritis (AA) model in rats showed that immunization with the mycobacterial hsp65 protects rats from AA. This protection is mediated by T cells recognizing the conserved 256–265 epitopes of the mycobacterial and the homologous rat hsp60 (see insert). Thus, bacterial hsp can induce self-reactive T cells that downregulate inflammatory processes. Since hsp60 is upregulated in inflamed joints, it appears possible that activated T cells recognizing this antigen may inhibit autoreactive T cells, for instance by the secretion of immunoregulatory cytokines (see text).

The insert shows the amino acid residues 256–270 of mycobacterial hsp65 and rat hsp60, respectively. Underlined are the 'core epitopes' recognized after immunization with either mycobacterial hsp65 or rat hsp60. While immunization with the mycobacterial hsp65 induces recognition of the highly cross reactive 256–265 epitope, immunization with the self-hsp60 induces recognition of the non-cross reactive epitope 261–270.

437–460 could protect NOD mice against diabetes.[31,53,54]

How could self-reactive T cells downregulate an inflammatory response? It has been proposed that cross reactive T cells might be cytotoxic for stressed synovial cells, which express high levels of self-hsp60.[43] Anti-idiotypic T-cell networks have also been proposed.[31] Another attractive possibility is downregulation of an inflammatory response via the secretion of anti-inflammatory cytokines produced by autoreactive T cells (Figure 2.1). It is well established in animal models of various infectious and autoimmune diseases that T-cell cytokine production is crucial for the outcome.[60] The same seems to be true for chronic inflammatory arthritides in humans.[2,61] One would very much like to know about the cytokine secretion patterns of those hsp60 256–270-specific rat T-cell lines. Unfortunately, in the rat model cytokine detection is not as easy as in mice or humans and therefore these data are not yet available (W van Eden, personal communication).

Whatever the mechanism, do these findings indicate that having some self-reactive T cells present is protective against autoimmunity? Do we all need our low-affinity self-reactive T cells to be regularly stimulated by cross reactivity with bacterial hsp? Earlier data seem to indicate that this might be the case. It was shown that a strain of rats normally resistant to induction of AA became susceptible when kept under germ-free conditions.[62] Resistance to arthritis induction was re-established upon infection with *Escherichia coli*.[63] On the other hand, susceptible strains remained susceptible irrespective of whether the animals were kept conventionally or germ free.[64] More data arguing *against* a protective effect of encountering bacterial antigens stem from two transgenic models of different diseases: rats transgenic for HLA-B27 and mice transgenic for a T-cell receptor recognizing an encephalitogenic epitope on myelin basic protein do not spontaneously develop disease when kept germ free. When kept conventionally, however, these animals develop disease spontaneously.[65,66]

Therefore, although it is now clear that molecular mimicry activating cross reactive T cells is not necessarily pathogenic and may even be helpful in some cases, the jury is still out on the question of whether the induction of immune responsiveness towards self-hsp is effective as a prophylactic or a therapeutic measure in experimental autoimmune disease. However, these difficult and sometimes contradictory findings from animal models have triggered intensive research on the human immune response to hsp.

ARTHRITIS AND THE HUMAN IMMUNE RESPONSE TO HSP

The human homologue of mycobacterial hsp65 is a mitochondrial protein called P1 or hsp60, which, as mentioned, shares 48% sequence identity with its mycobacterial counterpart. Early reports on immunological cross reactivity between mycobacterial hsp65 and human hsp60[8–12] and the upregulated expression of human hsp in inflamed synovium[58,67,68] induced a wave of research on the human immune response to hsp in various diseases. Some workers showed that cytotoxic T cells specific for bacterial hsp60 recognized and lysed stressed host cells in the absence of bacterial hsp peptides.[8–10]

The findings from the adjuvant arthritis model in rats (see above) motivated the search for hsp-reactive T cells in the synovial fluid from patients with rheumatoid arthritis (RA). T cells specific for the mycobacterial hsp65 were indeed found by various groups.[69–72] Similarly, T cells recognizing hsp65 were found in the synovial fluid of patients with Still's disease,[71] spondyloarthropathy,[71] psoriatic arthritis,[71] and juvenile chronic arthritis.[73,74] Some groups reported cross reactivity with the human hsp60,[11,73,74] but others did not.[72,75] When the hsp65 epitopes recognized by cross reactive T cells were mapped, it was found that self-hsp-reactive T cells responded to conserved epitopes that are shared between human hsp60 and mycobacterial hsp65.[11]

Similarly, in arthritis induced by *Salmonella* or *Borrelia burgdorferi*, strong T-cell responses towards bacterial hsp60 or hsp70 were described. However, there was no cross reactivity with the homologous human hsp, indicating that the T-cell response was directed against nonconserved epitopes.[72,76,77] In contrast, one group reported the isolation from the synovial fluid of a patient with *Yersinia*-induced reactive arthritis of a T-cell clone that recognized both the *Yersinia* and the human hsp60.[78] Interestingly, T-cell lines recognizing mycobacterial hsp65 were found significantly more frequently in leprosy patients with leprosy-associated arthritis than in leprosy patients without arthritis (W Cossermelli-Messina, AC Steere, and T Kamradt, manuscript in preparation).

Thus, hsp-recognizing T cells could be detected in the synovial fluid or the peripheral blood of patients with a variety of chronic inflammatory arthritides. Whereas these T cells specifically recognized microbial hsp in some cases, they displayed cross reactivity for human hsp in others. The latter findings leave one wondering whether the recognition of self-hsp is secondary to the recognition of bacterial hsp or vice versa. To complicate matters even further, Munk et al showed that self-hsp60-specific T cells could be isolated from healthy individuals who showed no signs of autoimmune disease;[10] Fischer et al found a high frequency of lymphocytes reactive with mycobacterial hsp65 in cord blood, thus making it unlikely that these cells need bacterial hsp for their elicitation.[79] Furthermore, Burmester et al found no significant response towards the mycobacterial hsp65 in peripheral blood mononuclear cells from patients with RA or other inflammatory joint diseases.[80] Another group found that the frequency of hsp65-reactive T cells was similar in the synovial fluid and the peripheral blood of patients with RA, thus arguing against a pathogenetic role for these cells.[81] What, then, is the significance of demonstrating pathogen-hsp-specific and/or self-hsp-specific cells in the blood or autoimmune lesions of patients?

Recently, de Graeff-Meeder and colleagues have examined prospectively the clinical significance of T-cell responses towards human hsp60 in patients with juvenile chronic arthritis (JCA).[82] They found self-hsp-reactive T cells predominantly, although not exclusively, in patients with a relatively mild and usually remitting course of the disease, namely patients with oligoarticular onset of JCA. These data seem to indicate that T cells which recognize self-hsp might not be harmful but may mediate protection or disease resolution. This is akin to the recent findings in AA[43] discussed above, and leaves similarly important questions to be answered: if these T cells are indeed protective, what is the mechanism? What are the self-hsp epitopes recognized by T cells from patients with a favourable clinical course of JCA? Which cytokines do these T cells produce upon activation? What is their phenotype and MHC restriction? Surely, these investigations must be under way and we can expect to learn much more about the functional significance of a T-cell response against self-hsp in chronic arthritis.

These findings seem to indicate that a T-cell response to self-hsp might be advantageous, but some recent data suggest that it might not: two recent publications described possible links between RA and hsp. Both started from the 'shared epitope' hypothesis.[83,84] This hypothesis (see Chapter 1) was based upon the observation that RA-associated HLA alleles share a conserved motif of basic charged amino acid residues in the third hypervariable region of their respective HLA-DRB1 molecules. This sequence can be one of the following (single letter code): QKRAA, QRRAA, or RRRAA. The fact that the dnaJ group of hsp of a variety of bacteria contains the QKRAA sequence[85] motivated Albani and co-workers to ask whether RA patients would generate an immune response against dnaJ or the QKRAA sequence. They found that peripheral blood mononuclear cells from patients with RA but not from controls proliferated in response to recombinant dnaJ. Furthermore, only RA patients but not healthy HLA DRB1*0401-positive controls responded to the synthetic peptide QKRAAYDQYGHAAFE.[86] Thus, the variant of the molecular mimicry hypothesis proposed by this group suggests cross reactivity between bacterial hsp and a human MHC class II molecule, instead of molecular mimicry between bacterial and human hsp. This is similar to the cross reactivity between the arthritogenic epitope of mycobacterial hsp65 and cartilage proteoglycan in the rat model of adjuvant arthritis (see above). The precondition for this hypothesis is that autoimmunity towards the 'shared epitope' should be pathogenetically important in rheumatoid arthritis. This is, of course, only one possible explanation of the 'shared epitope' hypothesis.

The other possible relationship between hsp and the 'shared epitope' in RA lies in antigen presentation. Auger and colleagues screened protein extracts from *E. coli* for binding to the QKRAA sequence. They found that bacterial hsp70 bound strongly to QKRAA and RRRAA. Furthermore, the constitutively expressed member of the human hsp70 group also bound to QKRAA and RRRAA. Finally, they showed that HLA-DRB1*0401 (containing the QKRAA sequence) and the human hsp70 co-precipitated in an immunoprecipitation assay.[87] Since hsp70 chaperones proteins and peptides into the lysosome,[23] this finding might have important consequences for antigen presentation: usually, HLA-DR molecules are synthesized in the endoplasmic reticulum (ER), where they associate with the invariant chain, which prevents peptides from occupying the peptide-binding groove. This complex leaves the ER and moves through the Golgi apparatus into endosomes. Here, the invariant chain is cleaved from the HLA class II molecules, which are then able to bind exogenous antigenic peptide encountered in the endosome, before being transported to the cell surface.[88] Pulse–chase experiments strongly suggested that in HLA-DRB1*0401 cells the HLA-DRβ chains bind to hsp70 in the ER and get chaperoned immediately into the lysosomes, bypassing the Golgi apparatus and the endosomes.[87] Possible consequences of this are (1) decreased expression of the HLA-DRB1 molecule at the cell surface; (2) impaired lysosomal transport of proteins containing the QKRAA or RRRAA sequences, due to competition with HLA-DR for hsp70 binding; (3) development of autoimmunity, due to increased presentation of hsp70 by HLA-DR; or (4) enhanced presentation of DRB1*0401 to T cells. The fact that HLA-DRB1*0401-positive individuals generate only weak T-cell responses against the QKRAA-containing Epstein–Barr virus gp110[89] may be due to impaired lysosomal transport, as outlined above. Although these possibilities are very interesting, one must not forget that the third 'shared epitope' sequence, QRRAA, did not show the same hsp70-binding pattern.[87]

SUMMARY

Hsp are expressed ubiquitously and show a high degree of sequence conservation between distantly related species. This, and the fact that almost any microbial infection will induce an immune response against (potentially cross reactive) hsp, has elicited great interest in the possible role of hsp in the induction or maintenance of autoimmune disease, including arthritides. The view of hsp as a link between infection and immunity was supported seemingly by the description of cross reactive T cells.[9] In its simplest form, this example of the 'molecular mimicry' hypothesis is that recognition of microbial hsp induces self-hsp-reactive T cells that are pathogenic. However, it is hard to explain why cross recognition of widely expressed molecules should lead to organ-specific autoimmune diseases such as arthritis or diabetes. This criticism could partly be answered by modifying the 'molecular mimicry' hypothesis to state that recognition of microbial hsp induces self-reactive T cells which recognize organ-specific antigens that share some homology with hsp. Examples of this are the cross reactivity between mycobacterial hsp65 and rat cartilage proteoglycan,[38] or the sequence homology between some HLA-DRβ molecules and bacterial hsp70.[86] Proof for this hypothesis would require convincing evidence that autoreactivity against the hsp-homologous self-proteins is indeed the pathogenic principle. This evidence is currently lacking for arthritides in humans. The modulation of antigen presentation by hsp[87] remains an interesting possibility, although its pathogenetic significance remains to be determined.

On the other hand, immunity to hsp has been implicated in protection from or downmodulation of autoimmune diseases, including arthritis.[43,54,82] The mechanisms by which these effects are exerted are currently unclear. For us, immunomodulation via anti-inflammatory cytokines seems the most attractive hypothesis (see Figure 2.1). As regards protective effects, the question of organ specificity can be answered with relative ease: self-hsp expression is upregulated in 'stressed' tissues such as inflamed joints, thus attracting the potentially beneficial self-hsp-reactive T cells. Why some patients with JCA make a beneficial T-cell response against self-hsp, while others do not, is currently unclear.[82] Animal models demonstrate that very subtle differences in the application of hsp can make the difference between a harmful and a beneficial self-hsp response. Taken together, the current evidence suggests that self-hsp-reactive T cells are a normally occurring population, which is regulated by a variety of ill-understood intrinsic and extrinsic factors. The initial idea that self-hsp-reactive T cells are the culprits for all autoimmunity was too simple. It is now clear that self-hsp-reactive

T cells are beneficial in some forms of arthritis, but one should carefully avoid regarding them as a panacea for autoimmunity, particularly because more data can be expected to accrue on exactly how these T cells mediate protection.

Although the hot air may finally have subsided, a fresh breeze is blowing through the field of hsp and arthritis.

ACKNOWLEDGEMENTS

This work was partly supported by the Senatsverwaltung für Wissenschaft und Forschung Berlin and the Deutsche Forschungsgemeinschaft (Bu 445). The authors wish to thank Dr NA Mitchison for critically reading the manuscript.

REFERENCES

1. Krause A, Kamradt T, Burmester G-R. Potential infectious agents in the induction of arthritides. *Curr Opin Rheumatol* 1996; **8**:203–9.
2. Burmester GR, Daser A, Kamradt T, Krause A, Mitchison NA, Sieper J, Wolf N. The immunology and immunopathology of reactive arthritides. *Annu Rev Immunol* 1995; **13**:229–50.
3. Kamradt T, Krause A, Burmester G-R. A role for T cells in the pathogenesis of treatment-resistant Lyme arthritis? *Molec Med* 1995; **1**:486–90.
4. Fujinami RS, Oldstone MB. Amino acid homology and virus: mechanism for autoimmunity. *Science* 1985; **230**:1043–5.
5. Burmester GR. Hit and run or permanent hit? Is there evidence for a microbiological cause of rheumatoid arthritis? *J Rheumatol* 1991; **18**:1443–7.
6. Burmester GR, Solbach W. Hit and run, hit and hide or permanent hit: why it is premature to dump Koch's postulates in rheumatic diseases. *J Rheumatol* 1992; **19**:1173–4.
7. Wucherpfennig KW, Strominger JL. Molecular mimicry in T-cell mediated autoimmunity: viral peptides activate human T-cell clones specific for myelin basic protein. *Cell* 1995; **80**:695–705.
8. Koga T, Wand-Württenberger A, DeBruyn J, Munk ME, Schoel B, Kaufmann SHE. T cells against a bacterial heat shock protein recognize stressed macrophages. *Science* 1989; **245**:1112–15.
9. Lamb JR, Bal V, Mendez-Sampeiro P, Mehlert A, So A, Rothbard J, Jindal S, Young RA, Young DB. Stress proteins may provide a link between the immune response to infection and autoimmunity. *Int Immunol* 1989; **1**:191–6.
10. Munk ME, Schoel B, Modrow S, Karr RW, Young RA, Kaufmann SHE. T lymphocytes from healthy individuals with specificity to self epitopes shared by the mycobacterial and human 65 kDa heat shock protein. *J Immunol* 1989; **143**:2844–9.
11. Quayle AJ, Wilson KB, Li SG, Kjeldsen-Kragh J, Oftung F, Shinnick T, Sioud M, Forre O, Capra JD, Natvig JB. Peptide recognition, T-cell receptor usage, and HLA restriction elements of human heat-shock protein (hsp) 60 and mycobacterial 65-kDa hsp-reactive T-cell clones from rheumatoid synovial fluid. *Eur J Immunol* 1992; **22**:1315–22.
12. Anderton SM, van der Zee R, Goodacre JA. Inflammation activates self hsp60-specific T cells. *Eur J Immunol* 1993; **23**:33–8.
13. Kaufmann SHE. Heat-shock proteins and the immune response. *Immunol Today* 1990; **11**:129–36.
14. Young RA. Stress proteins and immunology. *Annu Rev Immunol* 1990; **8**:401–20.
15. Lindquist SC. The heat shock response. *Annu Rev Biochem* 1986; **55**:1151–91.
16. Welch WJ. Mammalian stress response: cell physiology, structure/function of stress proteins, and implications for medicine and disease. *Physiol Rev* 1992; **72**:1063–81.
17. Lis J, Wu C. Protein traffic on the heat shock promoter: parking, stalling, and trucking along. *Cell* 1993; **74**:1–4.
18. Georgopoulos C, Welch WJ. Role of the major heat shock proteins as molecular chaperones. *Annu Rev Cell Biol* 1993; **9**:601–34.
19. Thomas PJ, Qu BH, Pedersen PL. Defective protein folding as a basis of human disease. *Trends Biochem Sci* 1995; **20**:456–9.
20. Flynn GC, Pohl J, Flocco MT, Rothman JE. Peptide-binding specificity of the molecular chaperone BiP. *Nature (Lond)* 1991; **353**:726–30.
21. Sargent CA, Dunham I, Trowsdale J, Campbell RD. Human major histocompatibility complex contains genes for the major heat shock protein HSP70. *Proc Natl Acad Sci USA* 1989; **86**:1968–72.
22. Flajnik MF, Canel C, Kramer J, Kasahara M. Evolution of the MHC: molecular cloning of

MHC class I from the amphibian *Xenopus. Proc Natl Acad Sci USA* 1991; **88**:537–41.
23. Terleckey S, Chiang H, Olson T, Dice JF. Protein and peptide binding and stimulation of in vitro lysosomal proteolysis by the 73 kDa heat shock cognate protein. *J Biol Chem* 1992; **267**:9202–9.
24. Suto R, Srivastava PK. A mechanism for the specific immunogenicity of heat shock protein-chaperoned peptides. *Science* 1995; **269**:1585–8.
25. Arnold D, Faath S, Rammensee H-G, Schild H. Cross-priming of minor histocompatibility antigen-specific cytotoxic T cells upon immunization with the heat shock protein gp96. *J Exp Med* 1995; **182**:885–9.
26. Bohen SP, Kralli A, Yamamoto KR. Hold 'em and fold 'em: chaperones and signal transduction. *Science* 1995; **268**:1303–4.
27. Hu J, Seeger C. Hsp90 is required for the activity of a hepatitis B virus reverse transcriptase. *Proc Natl Acad Sci USA* 1996; **93**:1060–4.
28. Buchmeier NA, Heffron F. Induction of *Salmonella* stress proteins upon infection of macrophages. *Science* 1990; **248**:730–2.
29. Jindal S, Dubani AK, Singh B, Harley CB, Gupta RS. Primary structure of a human mitochondrial protein homologous to the bacterial and plant chaperonins and to the 65-kilodalton mycobacterial antigen. *Mol Cell Biol* 1989; **9**:2279–83.
30. Matzinger P. Tolerance, danger, and the extended family. *Annu Rev Immunol* 1994; **12**:991–1045.
31. Cohen IR, Autoimmunity to chaperonins in the pathogenesis of arthritis and diabetes. *Annu Rev Immunol* 1991; **9**:567–89.
32. Kaufmann SHE. Heat shock proteins and autoimmunity: a critical appraisal. *Int Arch Allergy Immunol* 1994; **103**:317–22.
33. Wick G, Schett G, Amberger A, Kleindienst R, Xu Q. Is atherosclerosis an immunologically mediated disease? *Immunol Today* 1995; **16**:27–33.
34. Twomey BN, Dhillon VB, Latchman DS, Isenberg D. Lupus and heat shock proteins. In: *Stress Proteins in Medicine* (van Eden W, Young DB, eds.). Marcel Dekker: New York, 1996:345–57.
35. Mairesse N, Kahn MF, Appelboom T. Antibodies to the constitutive 73-kD protein. *Am J Med* 1993; **95**:595–600.
36. Pearson CM, Development of arthritis, periarthritis, and periostitis in rats given adjuvants. *Proc Soc Exp Biol Med* 1956; **91**:95–101.
37. Holoshitz J, Naparstek Y, Ben-Nun A, Cohen IR. Lines of T lymphocytes induce or vaccinate against autoimmune arthritis. *Science* 1983; **219**:56–8.
38. van Eden W, Holoshitz J, Nevo Z, Frenkel A, Klajman A, Cohen IR. Arthritis induced by a T-lymphocyte clone that responds to *Mycobacterium tuberculosis* and to cartilage proteoglycans. *Proc Natl Acad Sci USA* 1985; **82**:5117–20.
39. van Eden W, Thole JE, van der Zee R, Noordzij A, van Embden JD, Hensen EJ, Cohen IR. Cloning of the mycobacterial epitope recognized by T lymphocytes in adjuvant arthritis. *Nature (Lond)* 1988; **331**:171–3.
40. Billingham MEJ, Carney S, Butler R, Colston MJ. A mycobacterial heat shock protein induces antigen-specific suppression of adjuvant arthritis but is not itself arthritogenic. *J Exp Med* 1990; **171**:339–44.
41. Hogervorst EJM, Wagenaar JPA, Boog CJP, van der Zee R, van Embden JDA, van Eden W. Adjuvant arthritis and immunity to the mycobacterial 65 kD heat shock protein. *Int Immunol* 1992; **4**:719–27.
42. Yang X-D, Gasser J, Feige U. Prevention of adjuvant arthritis in rats by a nonapeptide from the 65-kD mycobacterial heat shock protein: specificity and mechanism. *Clin Exp Immunol* 1992; **87**:99–104.
43. Anderton SM, van der Zee R, Prakken B, Noordzij A, van Eden W. Activation of T cells recognizing self 60-kD heat shock protein can protect against autoimmune arthritis. *J Exp Med* 1995; **181**:943–52.
44. López-Guerrero JA, López-Bote JP, Ortiz MA, Gupta RS, Páez E, Bernabéu C. Modulation of adjuvant arthritis in Lewis rats by recombinant vaccinia virus expressing human 60 kDa heat shock protein. *Infect Immun* 1993; **61**:4225–31.
45. Hogervorst EJM, Schouls L, Wagenaar-Hilbers JPA, Boog CPJ, Spaan WJM, van Embden JDA. Modulation of experimental autoimmunity: treatment of adjuvant arthritis by immunization with a recombinant vaccinia virus. *Infect Immun* 1991; **59**:2029–35.
46. López-Guerrero JA, Ortiz MA, Páez E, Bernabéu C, López-Bote JP. Therapeutic effect of recombinant vaccinia virus expressing the 60-kd heat-shock protein on adjuvant arthritis. *Arthritis Rheum* 1994; **37**:1462–7.
47. Van den Broek MF, Hogervorst EJM, van Bruggen MCJ, van Eden W, van der Zee R, van

der Berg WB. Protection against streptococcal cell wall-induced arthritis by pretreatment with the 65-kD mycobacterial heat shock protein. *J Exp Med* 1989; **170**:449–66.
48. Thompson SJ, Rook GAW, Breley RJ, van der Zee R, Elson CJ. Autoimmune reactions to heat-shock proteins in pristane-induced arthritis. *Eur J Immunol* 1990; **20**:2479–84.
49. Kingston AE, Hicks CA, Colston MJ, Billingham ME. A 71-kD heat shock protein (hsp) from *Mycobacterium tuberculosis* has modulatory effects on experimental rat arthritis. *Clin Exp Immunol* 1996; **103**:77–82.
50. Ragno S, Winrow VR, Mascagni P, Lucietto P, Di Pierro F, Morris CJ, Blake DR. A synthetic 10-kD heat shock protein (hsp10) from *Mycobacterium tubcerulosis* modulates adjuvant arthritis. *Clin Exp Immunol* 1996; **103**:384–90.
51. Grippenberg-Lerche C, Toivanen A, Toivanen P. *Yersinia*-associated arthritis in rats: effect of 65 kDa heat shock protein, bovine serum albumin and incomplete Freund's adjuvant. *Clin Exp Rheumatol* 1995; **13**:321–5.
52. Zhang ZJ, Lee CSY, Lider O, Weiner HL. Suppression of adjuvant arthritis in lewis rats by oral administration of type II collagen. *J Immunol* 1990; **145**:2489–93.
53. Elias D, Markovits D, Reshef T, van-der-Zee R, Cohen IR. Induction and therapy of autoimmune diabetes in the non-obese diabetic (NOD/Lt) mouse by a 65-kDa heat shock protein. *Proc Natl Acad Sci USA* 1990; **87**:1576–80.
54. Elias D, Cohen IR. Peptide therapy for diabetes in NOD mice. *Lancet* 1994; **343**:704–6.
55. Kaufman DL, Clare-Saizier M, Tian J, Forsthuber T, Ting GSP, Robinson P, Atkinson MA, Sercarz EE, Tobin AJ, Lehmann PV. Spontaneous loss of T-cell tolerance to glutamic acid decarboxylase in murine insulin-dependent diabetes. *Nature (Lond)* 1993; **366**:69–72.
56. Tisch R, Yang X-D, Singer SM, Liblau RS, Fugger L, McDevitt HO. Immune response to glutamic acid decarboxylase correlates with insulitis in non-obese diabetic mice. *Nature (Lond)* 1993; **366**:72–5.
57. Anderton SM, van der Zee R, Nordzij A, van Eden W. Differential mycobacterial 65-kDa heat shock protein T-cell epitope recognition after adjuvant arthritis inducing or protective immunization protocols. *J Immunol* 1994; **152**:3656–64.
58. de Graeff-Meeder ER, Voorhosrs M, van Eden W, Schuurman H-J, Huber J, Barkley D, Maini RN, Kuis W, Rijkers GT, Zegers BJM. Antibodies to the mycobacterial heat shock protein are reactive with synovial tissue of adjuvant arthritis rats and patients with rheumatoid arthritis and osteoarthritis. *Am J Pathol* 1990; **137**:1013–17.
59. Kleinau S, Soderstrom K, Kiessling R, Klareskog LA. A monoclonal antibody to the mycobacterial 65 kD heat shock protein (ML 30) binds to cells in normal and arthritic joints of rats. *Scand J Immunol* 1991; **33**:195–202.
60. Liblau RS, Singer SM, McDevitt HO. Th1 and Th2 CD4+ T cells in the pathogenesis of organ-specific autoimmune diseases. *Immunol Today* 1995; **12**:34–8.
61. Feldmann M, Brennan FM, Maini RN. Role of cytokines in rheumatoid arthritis. *Annu Rev Immunol* 1996; **14**:397–440.
62. Kohashi O, Kutawa J, Umehara K, Uemura F, Takahashi T, Ozawa A. Susceptibility to adjuvant-induced arthritis among germfree, specific pathogen free and conventional rats. *Infect Immun* 1979; **26**:791–4.
63. Kohashi O, Kohashi Y, Takahashi T, Ozawa A, Shigematsu N. Suppressive effect of *Escherichia coli* on adjuvant-induced arthritis in germ-free rats. *Arthritis Rheum* 1986; **29**:547–52.
64. Bjork J, Kleinau S, Midtvedt T, Klareskog L, Smedegard G. Role of the bowel flora for development of immunity to hsp 65 and arthritis in three experimental models. *Scand J Immunol* 1994; **40**:648–52.
65. Taurog JD, Richardson JA, Croft JT, Simmons WA, Zhou M, Fernandez SJ, Balish E, Hammer RE. The germfree state prevents development of gut and joint inflammatory disease in HLA-B27 transgenic rats. *J Exp Med* 1994; **180**:2359–64.
66. Goverman J, Woods A, Larson L, Weiner LP, Hood L, Zaller DM. Transgenic mice that express a myelin basic protein-specific T-cell receptor develop spontaneous autoimmunity. *Cell* 1993; **72**:551–60.
67. Karlsson-Parra A, Soderstrom K, Ferm M, Ivanyi J, Kiessling R, Klareskog L. Presence of human heat shock protein (hsp) in inflamed joints and subcutaneous nodules of RA patients. *Scand J Immunol* 1990; **31**:283–8.
68. Boog CJP, de Graeff-Meeder ER, Lucassen MA, van der Zee R, Voorhorst-Ogink MM, van Kooten PJS, Geuze HJ, van Eden W. Two monoclonal antibodies generated against human hsp60 show reactivity with synovial membranes

of patients with juvenile chronic arthritis. *J Exp Med* 1992; **175**:1805–10.

69. Res PCM, Schaar CG, Breedveld FC, van Eden W, van Embden JDA, Cohen IR, de Vries RRP. Synovial fluid T-cell reactivity against 65 kD heat shock protein in early chronic arthritis. *Lancet* 1988; **ii**:478–80.
70. Holoshitz J, Koning F, Coligan JE, De Bruyn J, Strober S. Isolation of CD4⁻ CD8⁻ mycobacteria-reactive T lymphocyte clones from rheumatoid arthritis synovial fluid. *Nature (Lond)* 1989; **339**:226–9.
71. Gaston JSH, Life PF, Bailey LC, Bacon PA. In vitro responses to a 65-kilodalton mycobacterial protein by synovial T cells from inflammatory arthritis patients. *J Immunol* 1989; **143**:2494–500.
72. Gaston JSH, Life PF, Jenner PJ, Colston MJ, Bacon PA. Recognition of a mycobacteria-specific epitope in the 65-kD heat-shock protein by synovial fluid-derived T-cell clones. *J Exp Med* 1990; **171**:831–41.
73. De Graeff-Meeder ER, van der Zee R, Rijkers GT, Schuurman H-J, Kuis W, Bijlsma JWJ, Zegers BJM, van Eden W. Recognition of human 60 kD heat shock protein by mononuclear cells from patients with juvenile chronic arthritis. *Lancet* 1991; **337**:1368–72.
74. Life P, Hassel A, Wiliams K, Young S, Bacon P, Southwood T, Gaston JSH. Responses to gram negative enteric bacterial antigens by synovial T cells from patients with juvenile chronic arthritis: recognition of heat shock protein HSP60. *J Rheumatol* 1993; **20**:1388–96.
75. Gaston JSH, Life PF, van der Zee R, Jenner PJ, Colston MJ, Tonks S, Bacon PA. Epitope specificity and MHC restriction of rheumatoid arthritis synovial T-cell clones which recognize a mycobacterial 65 kDa heat shock protein. *Int Immunol* 1991; **3**:965–72.
76. Shanafelt M-C, Hindersson P, Soderberg C, Mensi N, Turck C, Webb D, Yssel H, Peltz G. T-cell and antibody reactivity with the *Borrelia burgdorferi* 60-kDa heat shock protein in Lyme arthritis. *J Immunol* 1991; **146**:3985–92.
77. Anzola J, Luft B, Gorgone G, Dattwyler RJ, Soderberg C, Lahesmaa R, Peltz G. *Borrelia burgdorferi* HSP70 homolog: characterization of an immunoreactive stress protein. *Infect Immun* 1992; **60**:3704–13.
78. Herrmann E, Lohse AW, Van der Zee R, Van Eden W, Mayet WJ, Probst P, Poralla T. Synovial fluid-derived *Yersinia*-reactive T cells responding to human 65-kDa heat-shock protein and heat-stressed antigen-presenting cells. *Eur J Immunol* 1991; **21**:2139–43.
79. Fischer HP, Sharrock CEM, Panayi GS. High frequency of cord blood lymphocytes against mycobacterial 65-kDa heat-shock protein. *Eur J Immunol* 1992; **22**:1667–9.
80. Burmester GR, Altstidl U, Kalden JR, Emmrich F. Stimulatory response towards the 65 kDa heat shock protein and other mycobacterial antigens in patients with rheumatoid arthritis. *J Rheumatol* 1991; **18**:171–6.
81. Fischer HP, Charrock CE, Colston MJ, Panayi GS. Limiting dilution analysis of proliferative T-cell responses to mycobacterial 65-kDa heat-shock protein fails to show significant frequency differences between synovial fluid and peripheral blood of patients with rheumatoid arthritis. *Eur J Immunol* 1991; **21**:2937–41.
82. de Graeff-Meeder ER, van Eden W, Rijkers GT, Prakken BJ, Kuis W, Voorhorst-Ogink MM, van der Zee R, Schuurman H-J, Helders PJM, Zegers BJM. Juvenile chronic arthritis: T-cell reactivity to human hsp60 in patients with a favorable course of arthritis. *J Clin Invest* 1995; **95**:934–40.
83. Gregersen PK, Silver J, Winchester RJ. The shared epitope hypothesis: an approach to understanding the molecular genetics of susceptibility to rheumatoid arthritis. *Arthritis Rheum* 1987; **30**:1205–13.
84. Winchester R, Dwyer E, Rose S. The genetic basis of rheumatoid arthritis: The shared epitope hypothesis. *Rheum Dis Clin North Am* 1992; **18**:761–85.
85. Van Asseldonk M, Simons A, Visser H, de Vos WM, Simmons G. Cloning, nucleotide sequence and regulatory analysis of the Lactococcus lactis dnaJ gene. *Intern Rev Immunol* 1993; **175**:1637–44.
86. Albani S, Keystone EC, Nelson JC, Ollier WER, La Cava A, Montemayor AC, Weber DA, Montecucco C, Martini A, Carson DA. Positive selection in autoimmunity: Abnormal immune responses to a bacterial dnaJ antigenic determinant in patients with early rheumatoid arthritis. *Nature Med* 1995; **1**:448–52.
87. Auger I, Escola JM, Gorvel JP, Roudier J, HLA-DR4 and HLA-DR10 motifs that carry susceptibility to rheumatoid arthritis bind 70-kD heat shock proteins. *Nature Med* 1996; **2**:306–10.
88. Cresswell P. Assembly, transport and function of MHC class II molecules. *Annu Rev Immunol* 1994; **12**:259–93.

89. Roudier J, Petersen J, Rhodes G, Luka J, Carson DA. Susceptibility to rheumatoid arthritis maps to a T-cell epitope shared by the HLA-Dw4 DRβ1 chain and the Epstein–Barr virus glycoprotein 110. *Proc Natl Acad Sci USA* 1989; **86**:5104–8.

3

Nonsteroidal anti-inflammatory drugs – gastroprotection – for whom exactly?

Gavin Lee and Peter Brooks

NSAIDS AND THE GASTROINTESTINAL TRACT

Nonsteroidal anti-inflammatory drugs (NSAIDs) are widely prescribed around the world; in 1993, 20 million prescriptions for NSAIDs were dispensed in Britain.[1] Around 20% of the population over the age of 65 have a current or recent NSAID prescription and NSAIDs are still prescribed extensively for noninflammatory rheumatic disease. They are now not only employed in rheumatic diseases but also in a variety of other painful conditions, such as postoperative pain, renal colic, and dysmenorrhoea, as shown in Table 3.1.

It is well recognized that the use of NSAIDs may result in unwanted gastrointestinal side-effects. These adverse events include gastric erosion, and peptic ulceration and its complications. The lower gastrointestinal tract may also be affected with ulceration, perforation, haemorrhage, increased protein loss, or a relapse of inflammatory bowel disease.[2,3] There is unfortunately a dissociation of pain and the presence of gastroduodenal lesions or ulcer complications. Whether this is due to the analgesic effect of the NSAID is unknown, but it may be associated with a clinically silent bleeding or perforated ulcer. The widespread prescription of NSAIDs[4] and extensive use of over-the-counter NSAIDs further amplifies the problem.[5]

Cross-sectional studies of upper gastrointestinal tract endoscopy among the users of NSAIDs demonstrate a prevalence of peptic ulcer of 14–31%.[6,7] In these studies, however, there is a possibility of overestimation of clinically relevant ulcers, as a number of silent lesions are identified and the clinical significance of these is still under debate.[8]

In a case–control study conducted by Savage et al[9] in a hospital setting consisting of 494 index patients, an odds ratio of 5:1 for haemorrhage or perforation of peptic ulcer in NSAID users was shown. The odds ratios for gastric and duodenal ulcer in this study were 5:9 and 4:9, respectively, although in previous studies NSAIDs were said to be associated with a risk of gastric but not of duodenal ulcer.[10,11] Langman et al[12] in Britain, conducted a case–control study of a group of 1144 patients

Table 3.1 Uses for NSAIDs
Inflammatory joint disease
Osteoarthritis
Soft tissue musculoskeletal disease
Renal and biliary colic
Peri- and postoperative analgesia
Colonic polyps and colon cancer
Alzheimer's disease

Table 3.2 Risk factors for gastrointestinal side-effects of NSAIDs

- Age
- Dose of NSAID
- Type of NSAID
- Multiple NSAIDs
- Previous history of peptic ulcer
- Co-prescription of corticosteroid
- Co-prescription of anticoagulant
- Co-morbidities
- Smoking
- Alcohol

aged 60 or older, presenting with acute upper gastrointestinal bleeding, and revealed that the use of nonaspirin NSAIDs was associated with an odds ratio of 3.5 for the ulcer complication. Earlier in the same year, Garcia Rodriguez and Jick[13] reported a study that had used a computer database of general practitioners to gather cases of upper gastrointestinal bleeding or perforation. They found that the adjusted estimate of relative risk of upper gastrointestinal bleeding with current use of NSAID use was 4.7.

Nonetheless, an accurate estimation of risk or incidence of NSAID-associated gastropathy is difficult. As pointed out in a meta-analysis by Bollini et al,[14] the design and the quality of the studies appeared to have a strong bearing on the outcome of the risk estimation reported. Higher risk estimates were found in case–control studies in comparison to cohort studies. Silent ulcers are not detected, and an underestimation of the incidence of peptic ulcers will result, unless endoscopy is carried out in all subjects.

Risk factors

There are a number of potential risk factors identified for the NSAID–gastrointestinal side-effects (Table 3.2). Fries et al[15] were one of the first groups to suggest that there might be differential effects of NSAIDs on the gastric

Table 3.3 Odds ratio and 95% CI for bleeding and perforation (Garcia Rodriguez and Jick) or acute gastrointestinal bleeding (Langman et al), and CSM rank order of serious reports of gut toxicity expressed per million prescriptions in the first 5 years of marketing

	CSM ranking	Garcia Rodriguez and Jick[13]		Langman et al[12]	
		Ratio	95% CI	Ratio	95% CI
Overall		4.7	3.8–5.7	4.5	3.6–5.6
Ibuprofen	1	2.9	1.78–5.0	2.0	1.4–2.8
Diclofenac	2	3.9	2.3–6.5	4.2	2.6–6.8
Naproxen	5	3.1	1.7–5.9	9.1	5.5–15.1
Ketoprofen	6	5.4	2.6–11.3	23.7	7.6–74.2
Indomethacin	*	6.3	3.3–12.2	11.3	6.3–20.3
Piroxicam	11	18.0	8.2–39.6	13.7	7.1–26.3
Azapropazone	12	23.4	6.9–79.5	31.5	10.3–96.9

*Not ranked by Committee on Safety of Medicines (CSM). Marketed before yellow card scheme.

mucosa. Data from the ARAMIS database have identified varying profiles of gastrointestinal reactions to NSAIDs similar to those shown in Table 3.3. It can be seen that the relative risk of a serious gastrointestinal side-effect of peptic ulceration and bleeding can vary significantly between NSAIDs.

Several other papers have been published in the past few years confirming the finding that some NSAIDs have a higher risk of inducing ulcer complication, such as bleeding and perforation.[9,12,13] However, in interpretation of these studies, care should be exercised to take into account the possibility of 'channelling' of a particular group of patients to a particular NSAID by the physician.[16] The degree of compliance may also be different between long-acting and short-acting drugs, with a different number of doses taken in a day. Despite this, there is accumulating evidence that some NSAIDs are less toxic to the gut than others, and this has recently been confirmed by a meta-analysis of these studies.[17] The recent demonstration that cyclooxygenase enzymes are of two types – a constitutive enzyme responsible for maintaining normal gastric and renal function (COX1), and an inducible form (COX2) seen in inflammation – has provided further data on NSAIDs and gastric injury. Moreover, NSAIDs have different COX1 : COX2 selectivity, with

Table 3.4 Cyclooxygenases (COX) 1 and 2: synthesis, function and inhibition

	COX1		**COX2**
Enzyme synthesis	Constitutive		Only after induction (IL-1, TNFα, lipopolysaccharide)
Function	Physiological protection of the stomach, regulation of platelet aggregation (TxA_2), peripheral vascular resistance (PGI_2), renal blood flow and intrarenal blood flow distribution (PGI_2, PGE_2), sodium excretion (PGE_2), and possibly ADH antagonism (PGE_2)		Proinflammatory prostanoids (PGE_2, PGI_2 and TxA_2) in fibroblasts and macrophages, and other cells
		Relative effect	
Inhibitors	← ← ← COX1 ← ← ← favours → → → COX2 → → →		
NSAIDs	Indomethacin		
	Aspirin		
	Piroxicam		
		Ibuprofen	
			Diclofenac
			Meloxicam
Glucocorticoids	No effect		Inhibition of enzyme synthesis

IL-1, interleukin-1; TNFα, tumour necrosis factor α; TxA_2, thromboxane A_2; PG, prostaglandin; ADH, antidiuretic hormone.

those agents having stronger COX1 inhibition being of higher risk for inducing adverse effects[18] (Table 3.4). Bateman[19] in fact has advocated that the use of NSAID should be based on these data, and if a NSAID is to be prescribed then the least toxic agent should be given.

Langman et al[12] have demonstrated the increase in risk of gastrointestinal toxicity with dose of NSAID, with an odds ratio of 2.5 for the low dose and up to 8.6 with the high dose. The study by Garcia Rodriguez and Jick[13] revealed a doubling of risk associated with those who use more than one NSAID simultaneously.

Langman et al[12] also found that the risk was generally greater for gastrointestinal toxicity during the first month among patients who had been taking a long-term NSAID. This might be due to higher than maintenance doses being employed in the initial period, or to the patients being more compliant in taking the drug compared to those long-term users. Withdrawal of those who suffer from side-effects of the NSAID from the group or population as time goes by might be an alternative explanation; or so-called 'mucosal adaptation' may be taking place. On the other hand, as pointed out by Bateman and Kennedy,[20] long-term users still develop gastrointestinal side-effects, and the risk involved in using NSAIDs does not disappear with prolonged exposure.

The other important risk factor is a history of peptic ulceration.[13,21–23] Not all lesions seen at endoscopy will progress and some of them can heal despite the continuation of NSAIDs, leading some investigators to suggest that erosions seen at an early stage of NSAID treatment may not be clinically significant. In contrast, Taha et al,[24] following up patients on NSAIDs with endoscopic examination up to 24 weeks, concluded that ulcers were more likely to develop in long-term NSAID users who had a mucosal erosion or evidence of infection with *Helicobacter pylori*.

A number of studies have been carried out concerning the role of *H. pylori* in NSAID-induced gastropathy, with both positive and negative associations being reported; no consensus has yet been reached.[23–25] There are data suggesting that *H. pylori* disrupts the hydrophobic mucosal surface, thereby causing it to lose its capacity to repel luminal acid.[26] Some other current data suggest that in healthy individuals *H. pylori* does not increase the risk of NSAID-induced gastroduodenal damage, although dyspeptic symptoms may be exacerbated in rheumatoid arthritis patients on NSAIDs. Nevertheless, NSAID use and *H. pylori* are two important but independent factors accounting for the refractoriness of the peptic ulcer, and the possibility of a synergistic relationship between the two should not be ignored, because of its potential therapeutic implication.[27]

Advanced age has been quite consistently shown to be associated with a high risk of development of a NSAID-related ulcer and its complications.[28] This is because age itself is associated with a significantly increased risk of peptic ulcer disease. Females have also been reported to have a higher incidence, but it should be noted that in a number of rheumatic diseases there is female preponderance that will in turn bias the cross-sectional studies. Moreover, as demonstrated by other studies, the risk of gastric bleeding while on NSAID treatment was actually higher in men.[22,29,30]

Alcohol is an irritant and a causative agent of gastritis and could also pose further risk for those taking NSAIDs. Savage et al[9] demonstrated a dose–response relationship between alcohol intake and complications of peptic ulcer. Smoking increased the risk of upper gastrointestinal bleeding by 40% in the group of patients reported by Garcia Rodriguez and Jick.[13] The use of corticosteroids and anticoagulants had an adjusted relative risk of 2.2 and 6.4, respectively, from the same study. Shorr et al[31] estimated a 13-fold increase in the risk of bleeding ulcer among the elderly (age >65) who were taking NSAID and anticoagulant concurrently.

The presence of debilitating arthritis is also reported to predict high risk in a subgroup of patients.[32] Janssen et al[23] studied this with the use of the Health Assessment Questionnaire

(HAQ), and revealed an association of borderline importance between HAQ score and current peptic ulcer disease. Moreover, the presence of liver and renal impairment, or cardiac failure will also increase the risk of toxicity to NSAIDs.

Finally, in relation to the upper gastrointestinal symptoms, studies have found these to be poor predictors of the presence of peptic ulcer.[23,33,34] It is, therefore, unwise to rely on symptoms to predict the presence of peptic ulcer, as it has been noted that a significant proportion of patients actually have silent peptic ulcers.

Pathophysiology

Figure 3.1 demonstrates those mechanisms involved in maintaining the integrity of the gastric mucosa. These can be classified into pre-epithelial, epithelial and postepithelial.[35,36] Pre-epithelial mechanisms consist of gastric mucus and the secretion of bicarbonate. The gastric mucus is secreted by mucus cells of the gastric mucosal epithelium and the gastric glands and is present in two phases – a soluble mucus phase and an insoluble mucus gel layer of about 2 mm in thickness. The bicarbonate ions are secreted by nonparietal gastric epithelial cells, and enter the mucus gel and contribute to the microenvironment immediately adjacent to the gastric mucosal cells. This unstirred layer of mucus gel slows the back diffusion of hydrogen ions from the lumen to the mucosal cell. The hydrophobicity and nonwettability of the mucosal surface have the ability to repel acid.[37] The gastric epithelial cell luminal surfaces and the intercellular 'tight' junctions resist the back diffusion of hydrogen ions, and is an important component of the mucosal defence. The mucosal blood flow is the postepithelial component of the mucosal defence. The maintenance of normal blood flow to the gastric mucosa is essential to maintain the integrity of the mucosa, due to its substantial oxygen requirement and high metabolic rate, and is critical for restitution after injury has occurred.[38]

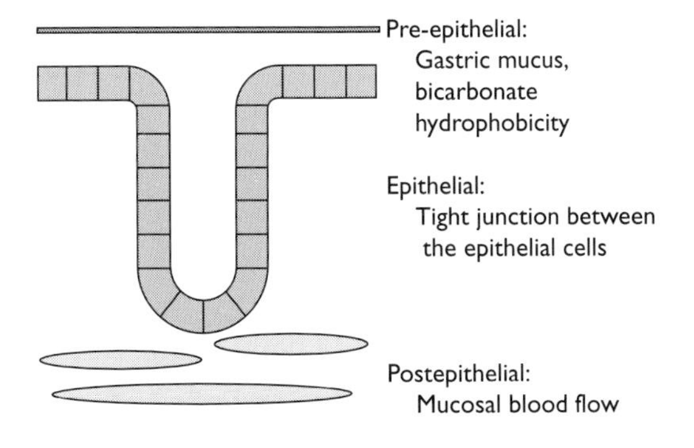

Figure 3.1 Mechanisms in the maintenance of the gastric mucosa.

Prostaglandins are involved in mucosal maintenance, since they inhibit acid secretion by blocking the action of histamine on parietal cells. Mucosal protection is also mediated through the increased secretion of gastric mucus and bicarbonate. Prostaglandins also have a role in maintaining mucosal blood flow and stimulating the rapid repair of disrupted epithelium. One of the enzymes involved in the production of the prostaglandins is the cyclooxygenase, which was recently noted to have two forms, the constitutive (COX1), responsible for maintaining renal and gastric function, and the inducible (COX2), found in inflammation. It is the COX1 enzyme that is responsible for the production of the cytoprotective prostaglandins in the gastric mucosa.

Nitric oxide also appears to be playing a role in gastric mucosal defence. The inhibition of the production of nitric oxide has been reported to reduce mucosal blood flow, causing leukocyte adhesion to the vascular endothelium with exacerbation of mucosal injury. As with prostaglandins, nitric oxide can be produced by either a constitutive NO synthase or an inducible NO synthase, and it is the constitutive enzyme responsible for the synthesis of nitric oxide that protects the gastric mucosa.[39]

The mechanisms of NSAID-induced mucosal injury can be divided into systemic and local effects, and both factors contribute, since parenteral and rectal administration of NSAIDs have been reported to cause gastrointestinal complications.[28] The systemic effect is mainly due to inhibition of the COX1 in the gastric mucosa, reducing the production of prostaglandin and resulting in a decrease of the thickness of the mucus gel layer, inhibiting the bicarbonate secretion and affecting mucosal blood flow. Inhibition of the cyclooxygenase also diverts arachidonic acid to the 5-lipo-oxygenase pathway and this may result in increased production of leukotrienes.[40] The role of leukotrienes in this situation is still controversial. In addition, the effect of NSAIDs on platelet function impairs haemostasis and may make bleeding more likely to occur.

Local application of NSAIDs will result in immediate damage to the gastric mucosa. The degree of damage depends on the solubility and the ionization constant (pK_a) of the specific NSAID.[40] The environment created by gastric acid promotes the production of a nonionized weak organic acid which will diffuse across the phospholipid membrane into the epithelial cell, where it will become ionized due to a higher intracellular pH. The acid will then be trapped, and these acidic NSAIDs will accumulate in relatively high concentration, and be presented to the gastric epithelial cells. Both the direct acid effect and the inhibition of cyclooxygenase will promote gastric damage.

Other possible mechanisms of injury by NSAIDs, not primarily due to cyclooxygenase inhibition, which have been reviewed by McCarthy,[41] include the elaboration of oxygen radicals, altered calcium fluxes and intracellular calcium concentrations, glutathione depletion, uncoupling of oxidative phosphorylation, and G-protein-mediated events. Recently NSAIDs were shown to induce apoptosis when applied to v-*src*-transformed chicken embryo fibroblasts and this may be of relevance in the maintenance of the integrity of the gastric mucosa.[42]

NSAIDs also have an effect on repair and healing of the gastric mucosa which includes the decrease of mucosal blood flow, affecting the formation of the mucoid cap. This is a requirement for cell migration into the denuded area and also causes inhibition of DNA synthesis following tissue injury, delay in the restoration of the disorganized subsurface architecture, and reduction in angiogenesis.[41]

It has been suggested that the depletion of prostaglandin only increases the susceptibility of the gastric mucosa to injurious agents such as gastric acid. However, the presence of gastric acid is not obligatory for the development of peptic ulcer in this circumstance; Janssen et al[43] pointed out that NSAIDs could induce benign ulcer disease in patients with achlorhydria.

It is reported that the mucosa will repair and heal despite the continued exposure to NSAIDs, leading to the suggestion that 'mucosal adaptation' occurs. Yeomans et al[37] claimed that there was a different degree of adaptation produced by various NSAIDs, and suggested that this might be due to the half-lives of the drug and the timing of the dose. Increased cell turnover resulting in a younger and more resistant epithelium, and the induction of cyclooxygenase are some of the suggested mechanisms mediating the adaptive process. The relevance of mucosal adaptation in healthy human subjects taking low-dose short-term NSAIDs has been challenged by Fenn,[44] because of the high-point prevalence of gastric mucosal damage and ulceration in screening endoscopic studies of arthritic patients.

GASTRIC PROTECTION

Different approaches have been employed in reducing the incidence of NSAID-induced gastropathy, based on the understanding of the pathophysiology. The concept of a balance of aggressive factors (acid and pepsin) and protective factors (the gastric mucosa) in the aetiopathogenesis of peptic ulcer led to trials of either the reduction of acid output (with the use of an H_2 receptor antagonist or proton pump inhibitor) or the strengthening of the mucosal defence (with

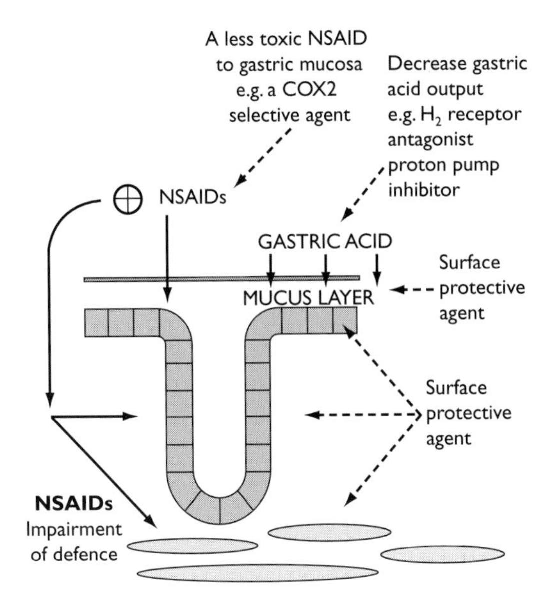

Figure 3.2 Gastric protection.

the use of a surface protective agent such as misoprostol) (Figure 3.2). As prostaglandins have been shown to be important in maintaining the gastric mucosa, the use of the prostaglandin analogue misoprostol has been extensively investigated. The potential role of nitric oxide in gastric mucosa protection has also attracted investigators to determine the possibility of its clinical application. Significant efforts are also being devoted to the design of less toxic NSAIDs, by manipulation of their pharmacokinetic and pharmacodynamic properties. This has led to the development of drugs such as nabumetone and a number of COX2 selective inhibitors such as meloxicam.

A different NSAID

In order to avoid direct topical contact between the gastric mucosa and NSAIDs, suppository and enteric coated agents were devised. Unfortunately, these have met with limited success only. It was shown that indomethacin oral capsules and suppositories caused a similar amount of gastric damage.[45] In addition to the important systemic effect of the drug, inhibiting the cyclooxygenase of the gastric mucosa, there is an indirect topical access to the mucosa via the biliary recycling of some NSAIDs and subsequent duodenogastric reflux.

Nabumetone is a new NSAID claimed to have a number of pharmacokinetic and pharmacodynamic properties that render it superior to the existing NSAIDs.[46,47] It is non-acidic in nature and it seems not to exhibit ion-trapping or to concentrate in the gastric epithelium. It is also a prodrug and is inactive as a cyclooxygenase inhibitor until it is metabolized by the liver. It is also claimed that, since its active metabolite (6MNA, 6-methoxy-2-naphthylacetic acid) does not have significant enterohepatic circulation, it will decrease the exposure of the intestinal mucosa to the drug. In animal studies, nabumetone exhibits COX2 selectivity, but this is less definite in human studies. The clinical experience of nabumetone has been reviewed by Richardson and Emery,[48] who report a significantly lower incidence of peptic ulcer, perforation and bleeding in nabumetone-treated patients (0.02–0.95%) in contrast to the previous studies with other NSAIDs (2–4% per year).

Meloxicam is a potent selective inhibitor of COX2, and has been tested in patients with osteoarthritis or rheumatoid arthritis. From the information available to date, it has a comparable efficacy to that of other NSAIDs with fewer gastrointestinal side-effects.[48] More studies and clinical experience need to be collected before its superiority in this regard can be confirmed. Other selective COX2 inhibitors, such as L-745,337, are under active investigation.[49]

As discussed above, the role of nitric oxide, which produces vasodilatation, improves mucosal blood flow, and interferes with neutrophil endothelial adhesion, has led investigators to conduct a study with a NSAID incorporating a nitroxybutyl moiety. Preliminary studies in animal models have demonstrated that the nitric oxide releasing NSAID shows a marked reduction of gastric toxicity and accelerates ulcer healing.[50,51]

Prostaglandin analogues

Graham et al in 1988 reported a double-blinded, placebo-controlled trial of prevention of NSAID-induced gastric ulcer with misoprostol.[52] They demonstrated that misoprostol significantly reduced the risk of gastric ulcer as detected by endoscopy in a dose-dependent manner. The protective effect on the development of duodenal ulcer was shown later by Geis et al.[53] In this study the incidence of duodenal ulcer among subjects on misoprostol 200 μg t.i.d./b.i.d. at 24 weeks was 1.4, while in the placebo group it was 9.7. White et al [54] showed a similar protective effect of misoprostol in their study. Hayllar [55] suggested that it was the acid-suppressing action of misoprostol that prevented the NSAID-related duodenal ulcer, while the additional protective actions such as increase in gastric mucosal blood flow and enhancement of repair mechanisms would account for its protective effect on the gastric mucosa.

Although there has been some doubt about the clinical significance of endoscopic studies relating to prophylaxis for NSAID-induced ulcer,[8] Silverstein et al[56] recently reported on the MUCOSA trial, which demonstrated that misoprostol produced a 40% reduction in gastrointestinal toxicity endpoints. In this extensive study, 25 of 4404 (0.57%) patients receiving misoprostol had serious ulcer complications, while there were 42 of 4439 (0.94%) patients receiving placebo who developed complications. However, there was a high premature withdrawal rate (39%) with significantly more patients in the misoprostol group stopping the drug because of diarrhoea, flatulence, and abdominal pain.

A fixed combination of diclofenac and misoprostol has been shown to have comparable clinical efficacy with other NSAIDs while maintaining a protective effect on the gastroduodenal mucosa in a group of osteoarthritic patients.[57,58] However, this type of combination drug produces significant side-effects, with more frequent abdominal pain and diarrhoea, 21% and 18%, respectively, in the study of Melo Gomes et al.[58] Moreover, Isdale and Wright[59] considered this fixed combination formulation to be not particularly useful in general, as it lost the flexibility of the dosage of either drug, and patients would be likely to have more side-effects from misoprostol if they required a higher dose of diclofenac for pain relief. Nevertheless, use of this combination drug might improve the compliance that is particularly important in elderly patients.

Although misoprostol has been shown to be effective in protecting against the NSAID-induced gastropathy, Taylor et al[60] demonstrated that misoprostol cannot totally restore the inhibition of gastric acid secretion induced by the administration of indomethacin. More important are the accompanying side-effects limiting its use and acceptance in patients.[61] Abdominal pain and diarrhoea have been reported in up to 40% of patients taking misoprostol and are dose-dependent. Misoprostol also has undesirable gynaecological effects such as bleeding, abdominal pain, and the risk of abortion in pregnant women.

H_2 receptor antagonist

Studies have shown that the H_2 receptor antagonist ranitidine has a limited role in preventing NSAID-induced gastric ulcer, although it is associated with a reduced prevalence of duodenal ulceration, as detected by endoscopy.[62,63] It has been questioned whether this was due to a dose that was inadequate for sufficient suppression of the gastric acid. Newer agents such as famotidine have been reported to be able to reduce the incidence of both gastric and duodenal ulcers, especially at a dose of 40 mg twice daily, in an endoscopic study of 6 months' duration.[64,65] Although nizatidine has been shown to reduce the ulcer occurrence in a high-risk group of patients, it did not significantly reduce the risk in the study group as a whole.[66] Further information is needed before we can accept that the newer H_2 receptor antagonists are of greater benefit.

Proton pump inhibitor

Omeprazole has been demonstrated to be superior in treating NSAID-induced peptic ulcer, and its efficacy unaffected by continuation of NSAIDs, when compared to H_2 receptor antagonists. However, information about its beneficial effect in preventing ulcer formation is limited. A study with 20 healthy subjects taking aspirin 2600 mg/day revealed that omeprazole 40 mg eliminated duodenal injury and also reduced gastric injury.[67] Ekstrom et al[68] demonstrated a reduction in frequency of gastroduodenal lesions and dyspeptic symptoms during NSAID treatment. However, it is difficult to draw any conclusion, in view of the small number of studies. Another drawback is the fact that the drug is relatively costly.

Other agents

Sucralfate, despite its use in preventing stress ulcer, has not been shown to be effective in preventing NSAID-induced gastric or duodenal ulcer.[69]

A study was conducted by Rodrigeuz de la Serna and Diaz-Rubio[70] using zinc acexamate, a drug that has antisecretory and mucosal protective activity. Among a group of patients with various rheumatic diseases and a previous history of peptic ulcer or intolerance to NSAIDs, there was a significant decrease in incidence of both gastric and duodenal ulcers in an endoscopic study conducted over a 4-week period.

IDENTIFICATION OF AT-RISK GROUP

Although studies have not always agreed in all aspects regarding the risk factors involved in the development of NSAID-induced gastropathy, some general guidelines can be developed from the information now available.

Clinical history is important in identifying the patients at risk. Most agree that age (>65 years) and the history of previous peptic ulcer are important factors, and that associated diseases not only increase the risk of toxicity but also render the patient less able to tolerate a significant bleed or an abdominal emergency. A debilitated state may also be a significant risk factor. The co-prescription of steroid or anticoagulant with NSAIDs is also important to consider. Although symptoms are poor predictors for the development of ulcer, it would be unwise to take persistent dyspeptic symptoms lightly, without careful investigation and exclusion of peptic ulceration.

Simple investigations may identify renal and liver function derangements that would affect the decision of NSAID treatment. Testing the stool for occult blood has a poor predictive value, and is not of any discriminating value in identifying a group at increased risk.

Use of endoscopy to screen the whole group of patients who are going to receive NSAIDs would not be practical or cost effective. However, once a patient has undergone endoscopy for persistent abdominal symptoms, and erosion is detected, then it would not be unreasonable to commence prophylactic drug treatment with misoprostol, omeprazole or a high-dose H_2 blocker.

Meddings et al[71] attempted to use sucrose as a permeability probe to identify gastric mucosal damage, and carried out both an animal study and a pilot study in humans. Greater mucosal damage was associated with a higher rate of sucrose excretion. This may be a useful attempt to develop a noninvasive method for the identification of a group at increased risk.

CONCLUSION

In order to provide gastric protection to patients receiving NSAIDs, universal co-prescription with anti-ulcer agents is definitely not cost effective. Bateman and Kennedy[20] estimated that if 20 million prescriptions for NSAIDs issued each year were each assumed to be for 1 month's treatment, then the cost of co-prescribing misoprostol or ranitidine would range from £200 million to £600 million, and it would cost £1 million to £3 million per life saved. Nevertheless, one should also consider morbidity in addition to mortality. Assessing the cost for the treatment of peptic ulcer disease, Levine[72] has estimated that the cost of preventive therapy with misoprostol is 6.5 times that of no treatment in a nonselected group of rheumatoid patients receiving NSAIDs. Gabriel et al[73] found that in patients over 60 years old, prophylactic treatment would be considered to be cost effective if the cost of a 3-month supply of misoprostol was equal to or below US$95, or the ulcer complication rate exceeded 1.5%. They also demonstrated that the cost effectiveness of misoprostol was sensitive to the cost of ambulatory care for the ulcer.[72]

Strategic NSAID drug prescribing by consideration of a series of questions will be helpful. Is a NSAID really required or can the pain be controlled by a simple analgesic? Can a less toxic NSAID be used, such as ibuprofen or a selective COX2 inhibitor? Can a lower dose of the NSAID be used? The above questions will be particularly important if the patient is in the high-risk group. Prophylactic treatment should be considered in patients older than 65 years of age who have a past history of peptic ulcer, or are taking steroids or anticoagulants, or have serious associated disease.

At the present time, misoprostol is the drug that has been shown to have the best protective effect on NSAID-induced mucosal damage, but is contraindicated in pregnant women. In order to save the cost in co-prescribing, it is important to investigate the clinical effectiveness of prescribing anti-ulcer agents for an initial 1 month only,[4,73] as there is some indication that there is a higher risk of complication during this initial peroid. Patient education is also important, to alert patients to the signs of gastrointestinal complications, and advise them to avoid other agents injurious to the gastric mucosa, such as cigarette smoking and alcohol.

REFERENCES

1. Prescription Pricing Authority. *Annual Report*. Prescription Pricing Authority: Newcastle upon Tyne, 1993.
2. Allison MC, Howatson AG, Torrance CJ, Lee FD, Russell RI. Gastrointestinal damage associated with the use of nonsteroidal anti-inflammatory drugs. *N Engl J Med* 1992; **327**:749–54.
3. Bjarnason I, Hayllar J, Macpherson AJ, Russell AS. Side effects of nonsteroidal anti-inflammatory drugs on the small and large intestine in humans. *Gastroenterology* 1993; **104**:1832–47.
4. Barrison I. Prophylaxis against non-steroidal induced upper gastrointestinal side effects. *Ann Rheum Dis* 1991; **50**:207–9.
5. Wilcox CM, Shalek KA, Cotsonis G. Striking prevalence of over-the-counter nonsteroidal anti-inflammatory drug use in patient with upper gastrointestinal haemorrhage. *Arch Intern Med* 1994; **154**:42–6.
6. Gabriel SE, Bombardier C. NSAID induced ulcers: An emerging epidemic. *J Rheumatol* 1990; **17**:1–4.
7. Larkas EH, Smith JL, Lipsky MD, Graham DY. Gastroduodenal mucosa and dyspeptic symptoms in arthritic patients during chronic non-steroidal anti-inflammatory drug use. *Am J Gastroenterol* 1987; **82**:1153–8.
8. Farr CM. NSAID-induced ulcers and prophylaxis: a reappraisal [editorial]. *J Clin Gastroenterol* 1993; **17**:187–8.
9. Savage RL, Moller PW, Ballantyne CL, Wells JE. Variation in the risk of peptic ulcer complications with nonsteroidal anti-inflammatory drug therapy. *Arthritis Rheum* 1993; **36**:84–90.
10. Duggan JM, Dobson AJ, Johnson H, Fahey P. Peptic ulcer and non-steroidal anti-inflammatory agents. *Gut* 1986; **27**:929–33.
11. Langman MJS. Epidemiologic evidence on the association between peptic ulceration and anti-inflammatory drug use. *Gastroenterology* 1989; **96**:640–6.
12. Langman MJS, Weil J, Wainwright P et al. Risks of bleeding peptic ulcer associated with individual non-steroidal anti-inflammatory drugs. *Lancet* 1994; **343**:1075–8.
13. Garcia Rodriguez LA, Jick H. Risk of upper gastrointestinal bleeding and perforation associated with individual non-steroidal anti-inflammatory drugs. *Lancet* 1994; **343**:769–72.
14. Bollini P, Garcia Rodriguez LA, Gutthann SP, Walker AM. The impact of research quality and study design on epidemiologic estimates of the effect of nonsteroidal anti-inflammatory drugs on upper gastrointestinal tract disease. *Arch Intern Med* 1992; **152**:1289–95.
15. Fries JF, Williams LA, Bloch DA. The relative

toxicity of non-steroidal anti-inflammatory drugs. *Arthritis Rheum* 1991; **34**:1353–60.

16. LeLorier J. Patterns of prescription of nonsteroidal antiinflammatory drugs and gastroprotective agents. *J Rheumatol* 1995; **22** (suppl 43):26–7.
17. Henry D, Lim L-Y, Garcia Rodriguez LA et al. Variability of risk of gastrointestinal complications with individual non-steroidal anti-inflammatory drugs: Results of a collaborative meta analysis. *Br Med J* 1996; **312**:1563–6.
18. Frolich JC. Prostaglandin endoperoxide synthetase isoenzyme: the clinical relevance of selective inhibition. *Ann Rheum Dis* 1995; **54**:942–3.
19. Bateman DN. NSAIDs: Time to re-evaluate gut toxicity. *Lancet* 1994; **343**:1051–2.
20. Bateman DN, Kennedy JG. Non-steroidal anti-inflammatory drugs and elderly patients. *Br Med J* 1995; **310**:817–18.
21. Begaud B, Chaslerie A, Carne X et al. Upper gastrointestinal bleeding associated with analgesic and NSAID use: A case–control study [letter]. *J Rheumatol* 1993; **20**:1443–4.
22. Hallas J, Lauritsen J, Villadsen HD, Gram LF. Nonsteroidal anti-inflammatory drugs and upper gastrointestinal bleeding, identifying high-risk groups by excess risk estimates. *Scand J Gastroenterol* 1995; **30**:438–44.
23. Janssen M, Dijkmans BAC, Lamers CBHW, Zwinderman AH, Vandenbroucke JP. A gastroscopic study of the predictive value of risk factors for nonsteroidal anti-inflammatory drug-associated ulcer disease in rheumatoid arthritis patients. *Br J Rheumatol* 1994; **33**:449–54.
24. Taha AS, Sturrock RD, Russell RI. Mucosal erosions in longterm non-steroidal anti-inflammatory drug users: Prediposition to ulceration and relation to *Helicobacter pylori. Gut* 1995; **36**:334–6.
25. Loeb DS, Talley NJ, Ahlquist DA, Carpenter HA, Zinsmeister AR. Long-term nonsteroidal anti-inflammatory drug use and gastroduodenal injury: The role of *Helicobacter pylori. Gastroenterology* 1992; **102**:1899–905.
26. Goggin PM, Marrero JM, Spychal RT, Jackson PA, Corbishley CM, Northfield TC. Surface hydrophobicity of gastric mucosa in *Helicobacter pylori* infection: effect of clearance and eradication. *Gastroenterology* 1992; **103**:1486–90.
27. Taha AS, Russell RI. *Helicobacter pylori* and nonsteroidal anti-inflammatory drugs: Uncomfortable partners in peptic ulcer disease. *Gut* 1993; **34**:580–3.
28. Henry D, Dobson A, Turner C. Variability in the risk of major gastrointestinal complications from nonaspirin nonsteroidal anti-inflammatory drugs. *Gastroenterology* 1993; **105**:1078–88.
29. Lanza LL, Walker AM, Bortinchak EA, Dreyer NA. Peptic ulcer and gastrointestinal haemorrhage associated with nonsteroidal anti-inflammatory drug use in patients younger than 65 years: A large health maintenance organization cohort study. *Arch Intern Med* 1995; **155**:1371–7.
30. Laporte JR, Carne X, Vidal X, Moreno V, Juan J. Catalan countries study on upper gastrointestinal bleeding. Upper gastrointestinal bleeding in relation to previous use of analgesics and nonsteroidal anti-inflammatory drugs. *Lancet* 1991; **337**:85–9.
31. Shorr RI, Ray WA, Daugherty JR, Griffin MR. Concurrent use of nonsteroidal anti-inflammatory drugs and oral anticoagulants places elderly persons at high risk for haemorrhagic peptic ulcer disease. *Arch Intern Med* 1993; **153**:1665–70.
32. Taha AS, Dahill RD, Lee FD, Russell RI. Predicting NSAID related ulcer: Assessment of clinical and pathological risk factors and importance of differences in NSAID. *Gut* 1994; **35**:391–5.
33. Bardhan KD, Bjarnason I, Scott DL et al. The prevention and healing of acute nonsteroidal anti-inflammatory drug-associated gastroduodenal mucosal damage by misoprostol. *Br J Rheumatol* 1993; **32**:990–5.
34. Janssen M, Dijkmans BAC, Sluys FA et al. Upper gastrointestinal complaints and complications in chronic rheumatic patients in comparsion with other chronic diseases. *Br J Rheumatol* 1992; **31**:747–52.
35. Scheiman JM. NSAID-induced peptic ulcer disease: a critical review of pathogenesis and management. *Dig Dis* 1994; **12**:210–22.
36. Soll AH, The pathogenesis of ulcers caused by nonsteroidal anti-inflammatory drug. In: *Nonsteroidal Anti-Inflammatory Drugs and Peptic Ulcer Disease* (Soll AH, moderator). *Ann Intern Med* 1991; **114**:307–19.
37. Yeomans ND, Skeljo MV, Giraud AS. Gastric mucosal defensive factors: the therapeutic strategy. *J Gastroenterol Hepatol* 1994; **9**:S104–8.
38. Bjorkman DJ, Kimmey MB. Nonsteroidal anti-inflammatory drugs and gastrointestinal disease: pathophysiology, treatment and prevention. *Dig Dis* 1995; **13**:119–29.

39. Hawkey CJ. Future treatments for arthritis: New NSAIDs, NO NSAIDs, or no NSAIDs? [editorial]. *Gastroenterology* 1995; **109**:614–16.
40 Hollander D. Gastrointestinal complications of nonsteroidal anti-inflammatory drugs: Prophylactic and therapeutic strategies. *Am J Med* 1994; **96**:274–81.
41. McCarthy DM. Mechanisms of mucosal injury and healing: the role of non-steroidal anti-inflammatory drugs. *Scand J Gastroenterol* 1995; **30** (suppl 208):24–9.
42. Lu X, Xie W, Reed D, Bradshaw WS, Simmons DL. Nonsteroidal anti-inflammatory drugs cause apoptosis and induce cyclooxygenase in chicken embroyo fibroblasts. *Proc Natl Acad Sci USA* 1995; **92**:7961–5.
43. Janssen M, Dijkmans BAC, Vandenbroucke JP, Biemond I, Lamers CBHW. Achlorhydria does not protect against benign upper gastrointestinal ulcers during NSAID use. *Dig Dis Sci* 1994; **39**:362–5.
44. Fenn GC. Review article: Controversies in NSAID-induced gastroduodenal damage – do they matter? *Aliment Pharmacol Ther* 1994; **8**:15–26.
45. Hansen TM, Matzen P, Madsen P. Endoscopic evaluation of the effect of indomethacin capsule and suppositories on the gastric mucosa in rheumatic patients. *J Rheumatol* 1984; **11**:484–7.
46. Blower PR. The unique pharmacologic profile of nabumetone. *J Rheumatol* 1992; **19** (suppl 36): 13–19.
47. Helfgott SM. Nabumetone: a clinical appraisal. *Semin Arthritis Rheum* 1994; **23**:341–6.
48. Richardson CE, Emery P. New cyclo-oxygenase and cytokine inhibitors. In: *Clinical Rheumatology: Innovative Treatment Approaches for Rheumatoid Arthritis* (Brooks PM, Furst DE, eds.). Baillière Tindall: London, 1995:731–58.
49. Chan CC, Boyce S, Brideau C et al. Pharmacology of a selective cyclooxygenase-2 inhibitor, L-745,337: A novel nonsteroidal anti-inflammatory agent with an ulcerogenic sparing effect in rat and nonhuman primate stomach. *J Pharmacol Exp Ther* 1995; **274**:1531–7.
50. Elliot SN, McKnight W, Cirino G, Wallace JL. A nitric oxide-releasing nonsteroidal anti-inflammatory drug accelerates gastric ulcer healing in rats. *Gastroenterology* 1995; **109**:524–30.
51. Wallace JL, Reuter B, Cicala C, McKnight W, Grisham MB, Cirinc G. Novel nonsteroidal anti-inflammatory drug derivatives with markedly reduced ulcerogenic properties in the rat. *Gastroenterology* 1994; **107**:173–9.
52. Graham DY, Agrawal WM, Roth SH. Prevention of NSAID-induced gastric ulcer with misoprostol: Multicentre, double-blind, placebo-controlled trial. *Lancet* 1988; **ii**:1277–80.
53. Geis GS, Stead H, WallemarkCB, Nickolson PA. Prevalence of mucosal lesions in the stomach and duodenum due to chronic use of NSAID in patients with rheumatoid arthritis or osteoarthritis, and interim report on prevention by misoprostol of diclofenac associated lesion. *J Rheumatol* 1991; **18** (suppl 28):11–14.
54. White R, Raskin JB, Jaszenski R, Teoh LS, Sue SO. Misoprostol and ranitidine in the prevention of NSAID-induced gastric and duodenal ulcer disease: A multicenter trial [abstract]. *Br J Rheumatol* 1992; **31** (suppl 2):180.
55. Hayllar J. Upper gastrointestinal tract. *Med J Aust* 1995; **162**:387.
56. Silverstein FE, Graham DY, Senior JR et al. Misoprostol reduces serious gastrointestinal complications in patients with rheumatoid arthritis receiving nonsteroidal anti-inflammatory drug: a randomized, double-blind, placebo-controlled trial. *Ann Intern Med* 1995; **123**:241–9.
57. Bolten W, Melo Gomes JA, Stead H, Geis GS. The gastroduodenal safety and efficacy of the fixed combination of diclofenac and misoprostol in the treatment of osteoarthritis. *Br J Rheumatol* 1992; **31**:753–8.
58. Melo Gomes JA, Roth SH, Zeeh J, Bruyn GAW, Woods EM, Geis GS. Double-blind comparison of efficacy and gastroduodenal safety of diclofenac/misoprostol, piroxicam, and naproxen in the treatment of osteoarthritis. *Ann Rheum Dis* 1993; **52**:881–5.
59. Isdale A, Wright V. Misoprostol/NSAID fixed combinations: help or hindrance in clinical practice? *Drug Saf* 1995; **12**:291–8.
60. Taylor SD, Chey WY, Scheiman JM. Acid secretion during indomethacin therapy: effect of misoprostol. *J Clin Gastroenterol* 1995; **20**:131–5.
61. Gabriel SE, Campion ME, O'Fallon WM. Patient preferences for nonsteroidal anti-inflammatory drug related gastrointestinal complications and their prophylaxis. *J Rheumatol* 1993; **20**:358–61.
62. Ehsanullah RSB, Page MC, Tildesley G, Wood JR. Prevention of gastroduodenal damage induced by nonsteroidal anti-inflammatory drugs: controlled trial of ranitidine. *Br Med J* 1988; **297**:1017–21.

63. Robinson MG, Griffin JW, Bowers J, Kogan FJ, Kogut DG, Lanza FL, Warner CW. Effect of ranitidine gastroduodenal mucosal damage induced by nonsteroidal anti-inflammatory drugs. *Dig Dis Sci* 1989; **34**:424–8.
64. Taha AS, Hudson N, Hawkey CJ et al. Famotidine for the prevention of gastric and duodenal ulcers caused by non-steroidal anti-inflammatory drugs. *New Engl J Med* 1996; **334**:1435–6.
65. Hudson N, Taha AS, Russell RI et al. High dose famotidine as healing and maintenance treatment for nonsteroidal anti-inflammatory drug-associated gastroduodenal ulceration [abstract]. *Gastroenterology* 1995; **108** April:A117.
66. Levine LR, Cloud ML, Enas NH. Nizatidine prevents peptic ulceration in high-risk patients taking nonsteroidal anti-inflammatory drugs. *Arch Intern Med* 1993; **153**:2449–54.
67. Scheiman JM, Behler EM, Loeffler KM, Elta GH. Omeprazole ameliorates aspirin-induced gastroduodenal injury. *Dig Dis Sci* 1994; **39**:97–103.
68. Ekstrom P, Carling L, Wetterhus S, Wingren PE. Omeprazole reduces the frequency of gastroduodenal lesions and dyspeptic symptoms during NSAID treatment [abstract]. *Gastroenterology* 1995; **108**:A87.
69. Agrawal NM, Graham DY, White RH, Germain B, Brown JA, Stromatt SC. Misoprostol compared with sucralfate in the prevention of nonsteroidal anti-inflammatory drug-induced gastric ulcer: a randomized, controlled trial. *Ann Intern Med* 1991; **115**:195–200.
70. Rodriguez de la Serna A, Diaz-Rubio M. Multicenter clinical trial of zinc acexamate in the prevention of nonsteroidal anti-inflammatory drug induced gastroenteropathy. *J Rheumatol* 1994; **21**:927–33.
71. Meddings JB, Sutherland LR, Byles NI, Wallace JL. Sucrose: A novel permeability marker for gastroduodenal disease. *Gastroenterology* 1993; **104**:1619–26.
72. Levine JS. Misoprostol and nonsteroidal anti-inflammatory drugs: a tale of effects, outcomes and costs [editorial]. *Ann Intern Med* 1995; **123**(4):309–10.
73. Gabriel SE, Campion ME, O'Fallon WM. A cost–utility analysis of misoprostol prophylaxis for rheumatoid arthritis patients receiving nonsteroidal anti-inflammatory drugs. *Arthritis Rheum* 1994; **37**:333–41.
74. Gabriel SE, Jaakkimainen RL, Bombardier C. The cost-effectiveness of misoprostol for non-steroidal anti-inflammatory drug-associated adverse gastrointestinal events. *Arthritis Rheum* 1993; **36**:447–59.
75. Stalmkowicz R, Rachmilewitz D. NSAID-induced gastroduodenal damage: Is prevention needed? A review and meta-analysis. *J Clin Gastroenterol* 1993; **17**:238–43.

4

Should methotrexate really be used as a second-line drug in the management of rheumatoid arthritis?

Roger D Sturrock

INTRODUCTION

Methotrexate (MTX) has become the 'gold standard' second-line drug for the treatment of rheumatoid arthritis (RA) in the last 10 years and is now widely used by rheumatologists as the drug of choice for the treatment of RA in the early phases of the disease. The rationale for this remarkable popularity of MTX is based on the perception that it has a fast onset of action, is well tolerated despite being a cytotoxic agent, and shows a lower drop-out rate in patients when compared with other second-line drugs. There is some evidence that MTX slows the rate of radiological progression of RA. All these features provide compelling reasons for the drug's current number one position in the rheumatologist's armamentarium. The object of this review is to revisit some of the data which have led to this conclusion and to assess whether the current status and position of MTX in the therapy of RA is justified. First, it would be helpful to define what is currently understood by a second-line drug and to consider the terms 'symptom-modifying antirheumatic drug' (SMARD) and 'disease-controlling antirheumatic therapy' (DC-ART).

Traditionally first-line drug therapy has been considered to encompass the use of non-steroidal anti-inflammatory drugs (NSAIDs) and analgesic agents for the treatment of RA.[1] Second-line drugs are those which are used in the face of continuing active disease and, in contrast to NSAIDs, have a slow onset of action (months rather than weeks), and have the effects of lowering the erythrocyte sedimentation rate (ESR) and the levels of C-reactive protein and rheumatoid factor levels.[2] They also improve functional status, and some, such as injectable gold, slow down the rate of radiological progression of RA.[3] These drugs are associated with significant toxicity and their precise mode of action in RA is unknown, although there is a large body of literature reporting many and varied effects on the immune system.[4] At present there is no substantial evidence that they fundamentally alter the underlying disease process in RA or that they are uniformly disease-controlling drugs (DC-ARTs) and hence the term SMARD has been used for many of the members of this group of drugs.[5]

The term DC-ART has been defined by the World Health Organization[6] as a drug that changes the course of RA by at least 1 year, as evidenced by a sustained improvement in physical function, decreased inflammatory synovitis, and a slowing or prevention of structural joint damage. If this strict definition is used, then the only drugs that even conceivably fall into this category are gold, cyclophosphamide and possibly MTX and sulphasalazine.

Table 4.1 Interactions of drugs with methotrexate

Interacting drug	Effect
Penicillins NSAIDs Probenecid	Reduced renal clearance of MTX
Cotrimoxazole/ Trimethoprim	Megaloblastic pancytopenia
Fluorouracil	Skin blistering and necrosis at site of topical application
Nonabsorbable antibiotics (vancomycin, neomycin, nystatin, polymyxin B)	Decreased absorption of MTX (up to 50%)

Table 4.2 Toxic effects of methotrexate

Effect	Comment
Hepatotoxicity	The long-term problem of liver fibrosis
Infections	Increased incidence of bacterial infection and problems with surgical sepsis
Pneumonitis	May occur early in the course of therapy
Osteopathy	Potential problems with long-term osteomalacia
Teratogenesis	The drug can only be used in premenopausal women only if they are using adequate contraceptive measures
Carcinogenesis	This is a theoretical risk, but appears not to be a clincal problem to date

PHARMACOLOGY OF METHOTREXATE

This review is not the place for a detailed description of the pharmacology of MTX, but it is important to discuss the principal modes of action of the drug, as this will enable a proper perspective to be put on the 'cost/benefit ratio' to be achieved by its use in the treatment of RA. It is essential to remember that MTX belongs to the class of cytotoxic drugs and its primary action is as a dihydrofolate reductase inhibitor, leading to an inhibition of the activity of thymidylate synthetase which results in the impairment of DNA synthesis and cell death.[7] As a result, it has a toxic effect on T-cell,[8] B-cell[9] and polymorphonuclear leukocyte function.[10] It inhibits the growth of fibroblasts and osteoblasts in culture,[11,12] and has variable effects on cytokine levels.[13–17] Once absorbed, MTX is 50% protein bound and is found in high concentrations in synovial membrane and in cortical and trabecular bone in RA patients.[18] Excretion is primarily as the parent compound via the kidneys by glomerular filtration and active tubular transport. Drug interactions are well documented[7] (Table 4.1) and in particular NSAIDs can interfere with the renal clearance of MTX and may be associated with life-threatening side-effects.[19] Antifolate agents also enhance the potential of MTX to cause haematological disorders; broad-spectrum antibiotics such as tetracycline and chloramphenicol can decrease its absorption from the gut.[20]

TOXICITY

Much has been made of the minimal toxicity of low-dose MTX in the long-term treatment of RA,[21,22] despite its potential for causing immunosuppression, blood dyscrasias and teratogenesis. These side-effects can be explained by its antifolate properties, but there are many other toxic manifestations that are still poorly understood. The potential toxic effects of MTX have been extensively reviewed,[23] but there are some toxic effects that have caused most concern and distinguish MTX from the other 'standard' second-line drugs. These are listed in Table 4.2.

Hepatotoxicity

The potential for MTX to cause liver damage has been well recognized for many years by dermatologists who have used the drug to treat severe psoriasis.[24] However, the precise incidence of clinically significant liver fibrosis in RA patients treated with low-dose weekly MTX is uncertain. A large retrospective survey of 259 patients treated with MTX for inflammatory arthritis, and who had undergone serial liver biopsies over a period of 8 years, found that 2.9% of RA patients had fibrotic liver disease that could not be predicted by abnormal liver function tests.[25] This is in contrast to a smaller prospective study, which demonstrated that minor changes in liver histology occurred in 52% of 27 patients, and correlated with elevation of liver enzymes. Risk factors for liver pathology were obesity, alcohol intake, and dose and duration of MTX.[26] The same group of rheumatologists undertook a more recent study, using light and electron microscopic analysis of serial liver biopsies of 27 RA patients followed over a mean period of 8.2 years, with a mean of 6.3 liver biopsies per patient. Surprisingly, there was little evidence for significant progression of the disease found by liver histology, and no clinically significant deterioration of liver function occurred.[27] However, case reports of severe liver fibrosis in RA patients on MTX can be found in the literature,[28] and a large review of MTX and liver toxicity suggested that the incidence of the progression of liver disease was 28%, although this figure was much lower in RA (approximately 3%).[29] Nevertheless, the long-term consequences of continued low-dose MTX treatment on the liver in RA remain unknown.

Infections

One of the characteristics of cytotoxic drugs is their suppression of the immune system, with the resultant increased risk of opportunistic infection. There is an increasing trend to use higher dosages of MTX in RA, at least in the early phase of treatment, and perhaps without the consideration that RA patients have an increased incidence of infection in the first instance, and this may be greatly enhanced by MTX. Case reports of opportunistic infections with *Pneumocystis carinii* and fungi[30,31] in low-dose MTX treatment are well documented and the possibility of predisposing RA patients to a recrudescence of Epstein–Barr virus (EBV) infection has been debated.[32] A more disturbing report is of the increased risk of postoperative joint infections in patients undergoing elective total joint arthroplasty, if MTX is continued throughout the perioperative period.[33] The practice in my unit is to stop MTX administration 2 weeks prior to any surgery and to restart the drug when the stitches are out and the surgical wound has healed. These reports emphasize the need for continued vigilance when MTX is used in RA, and the need to maintain a high index of suspicion of infection when patients develop unexpected symptoms.

Pneumonitis

Although MTX causes an increased risk of lung infection, it is also associated with acute pneumonitis and chronic pulmonary fibrosis (methotrexate lung). The acute pneumonitis can be difficult to distinguish from adult respiratory distress syndrome (ARDS) and is characterized by the development of a cough with rapidly progressing respiratory failure and diffuse reticular interstitial infiltrates[34,35] (Figure 4.1). The onset of pneumonitis is not dose related[35] and can occur early in the course of treatment, but pre-existing pulmonary disease does not appear to increase the risk of pneumonitis.[36] This suggests that MTX hypersensitivity is the predominant mechanism involved. Long-term lung fibrosis remains an anxiety, but this occurs more frequently in cancer patients treated with higher doses of MTX.[37] The overall frequency of pneumonitis with low-dose MTX in RA is difficult to

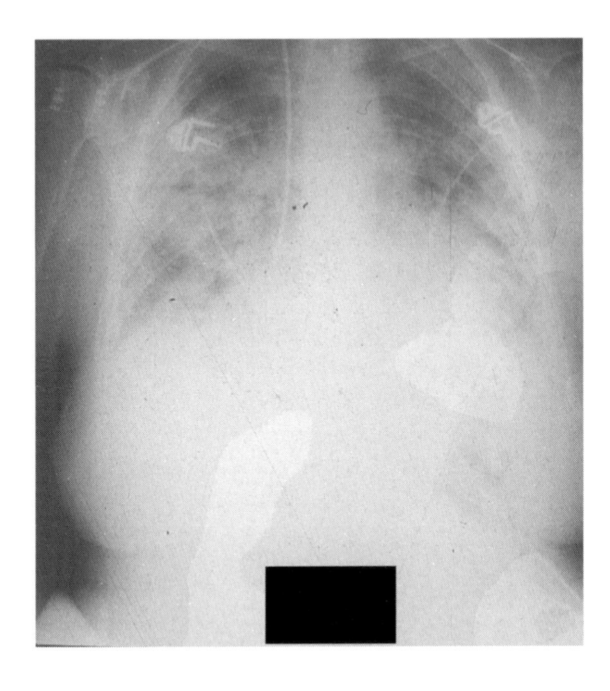

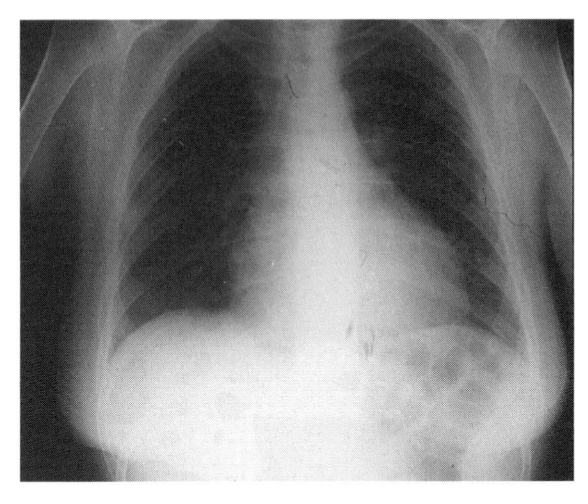

Figure 4.1 Methotrexate lung in a 32-year-old female patient before (left) and after (right) treatment with high dose steroids. She had been on 7.5 mg of methotrexate for 3 months prior to this complication.

estimate, but figures of 3–7% and 0.3–11.6% have been quoted.[38,39]

Osteopathy

MTX can inhibit osteoblast function,[12] and osteopathy has been observed in children treated with high-dose MTX for leukaemia.[40] As yet there are no long-term follow-up studies on RA patients to determine whether osteoporosis and osteomalacia are likely to be significant problems with low dose MTX, although a study of low-dose MTX in rats has shown that bone formation and bone were significantly reduced in the MTX-treated animals.[41]

Teratogenesis

The cytotoxic group of drugs vary in their potential for teratogenesis, but MTX is definitely teratogenic[42] and can cause impaired spermatogenesis, chromosomal abnormalities, and single-gene mutations.[43] The latter effects should be taken into consideration when boys and young men are treated with MTX . Women of childbearing age must take adequate contraceptive measures while on MTX.[42]

Carcinogenesis

There is obvious concern that MTX may be associated with an increased long-term risk of malignancy, but the evidence for this to date is at best tenuous. The problem is that RA itself is associated with an increased risk of lymphoma.[43] However, leukaemia[44] and reversible lymphomas associated with EBV infection[45] have been reported in MTX-treated RA patients. Long-term carcinogenesis must therefore remain a concern in young patients who embark on long-term MTX treatment for their inflammatory joint disease.

REVIEW OF CLINICAL TRIALS

The success of MTX in the treatment of psoriasis and the observation that patients with psoriatic arthritis noted an improvement in their joint symptoms led to a spate of reports in the 1970s of its successful use in inflammatory joint disease.[46–48] Hoffmeister can be credited with the first report of the long-term assessment of the effects of MTX in the treatment of RA.[49] He described the effects of MTX on 78 RA patients followed up for 15 years and noted that 58% showed marked improvement or complete remission without the occurrence of any serious toxicity. There then followed the publication of a number of placebo-controlled double-blind trials,[50–52] which clearly showed that MTX was superior to placebo in improving the standard clinical parameters such as swollen joint count, grip strength, and duration of morning stiffness. Significant falls in the ESR and level of rheumatoid factor together with a rise in haemoglobin level were reported. Long-term follow-up studies with low-dose weekly MTX showed that MTX had a steroid-sparing effect and that life table analysis projected that 63% of patients would receive therapy for 6 years.[53]

Comparative trials with other second-line agents have been flawed by the small numbers of patients in the comparator groups, but Felson and colleagues, in two meta-analysis studies of trials that in total included almost 5000 patients, demonstrated that MTX performed well in terms of toxicity, drop-out rate, and efficacy.[54,55] Little difference could be found between injectable gold, D-penicillamine and sulphasalazine as far as efficacy was concerned, although injectable gold was found to be the most toxic in the short term. A more recent, prospective, 5-year multicentre study that compared MTX with auranofin reported marked improvement in 71% of MTX treated patients, with 64% still taking MTX at the end of 5 years.[56]

Methotrexate has been shown to have a positive effect on physical, social, and emotional function in RA,[57] but its effects on disease progression as measured by radiology are not so clearcut. Several studies have suggested that MTX may slow down the rate of radiological progression of RA,[58,59] but again the number of patients available for analysis was small. Alarcon and co-workers undertook a meta-analysis of available and analysable radiological studies and did not find any significant differences in the erosion scores when MTX was compared to other disease-modifying antirheumatic drugs (SMARDs), with gold salts being superior to MTX.[60] A subsequent study by Alarcon and colleagues of the Cooperative Systematic Studies of auranofin vs MTX and a combination of the two found that erosion scores worsened in all three groups, but that the group receiving auranofin only deteriorated significantly from baseline.[61] Clearly, further studies should be carried out in early RA to determine whether MTX significantly affects radiological progression of disease, perhaps with the use of novel methods of scoring the erosion rate[62] and more sensitive techniques such as magnetic resonance imaging.

SHOULD MTX BE USED AS A SECOND-LINE DRUG? ITS PLACE IN THERAPY

There is no doubt that MTX has the properties of a second-line antirheumatic drug and fulfills the criteria of a SMARD. Moreover, it has 'added value' in both dual and triple combination therapy.[63,64] Together with its rapid onset of action and relatively low long-term drop-out rate, it appears to be an attractive option as the preferred second-line drug for the treatment of RA. Rheumatologists are undergoing a philosophical change in their approach to drug therapy in RA, in that there has been a challenge[65] to the 'traditional' pyramidal approach to drug usage, with NSAIDs being the first line in treatment, followed by a subsequent gradual introduction of second-line drugs, and with cytotoxics and immunomodulators such as cyclosporine being reserved for use in resistant cases. Healey and Wilske[65] propose the early use of combination therapy – a theme that is echoed by Fries[66] in his description of the 'sawtooth' strategy. There is certainly some evidence that the early introduction of second-line drugs in 238 RA patients studied by Van der Heide and colleagues[67] was of clinical benefit in the group of patients who received this treatment, although radiological erosive scores deteriorated at the same rate in both the second-line and non-second-line groups. Should MTX be used early in RA? The current body of knowledge suggests that this is a reasonable strategy, but I personally would have some reservations about this policy until we know more about the long-term toxicity of low-dose MTX, especially in younger patients. Can MTX be considered as a potential DC-ART? The evidence for this is not available at present, but carefully conducted controlled trials in early RA may give the answer. It remains to be seen whether any of the currently available second-line agents fulfil all the criteria demanded by this definition.[6]

Methotrexate is certainly a very interesting drug as far as rheumatologists are concerned. It is potentially the best drug we have currently available for the treatment of RA, but we would do well to heed the words of William Heberden[68] before making too precipitous a judgement relating to its role in rheumatology:

The difficulty of ascertaining the powers of medicines, and of distinguishing their real effects from the changes wrought in the body by other causes, must have been felt by every physician: and no aphorism of Hippocrates holds truer to this day, than that in which he laments the length of time necessary to establish medical truths, and the danger, unless caution be used, of our being misled even by experience.

REFERENCES

1. Porter DR, Sturrock RD. Medical management of rheumatoid arthritis. *Br Med J* 1993; **307**:425–8.
2. Capell H, Brzeski M. Slow drugs: slow progress? Use of slow activating antirheumatic drugs (SAARDs) in rheumatoid arthritis. *Ann Rheum Dis* 1992; **51**:424–9.
3. Pullar T, Capell H. A rheumatological dilemma: is it possible to alter the course of rheumatoid arthritis? Can we answer the question? *Ann Rheum Dis* 1985; **44**:134–40.
4. Olsen NJ, Callahan LF, Pincus T. Immunologic studies of rheumatoid arthritis patients treated with methotrexate. *Arthritis Rheum* 1987; **30**:481–8.
5. Edmonds J. DC-ART: the concept. *J Rheumatol* 1994; **41**:3–5.
6. Paulus HE, Bulpitt KJ. DC ART classification: review of relevant clinical studies – Review. *J Rheumatol* 1994; **41**:8–20.
7. Baggott JE, Morgan SL, Ha TS et al. Antifolates in rheumatoid arthritis: a hypothetical mechanism of action. *Clin Exp Rheumatol* 1993; **11**:S101–5.
8. Ridge SC, Ferguson KM, Rath N et al. Methotrexate in mononuclear cells derived from normal and adjuvant arthritic rats. *J Rheumatol* 1988; **15**:1193–7.
9. Olsen NY, Callahan LF, Pincus T. Immunological studies of rheumatoid arthritis patients treated with methotrexate. *Arthritis Rheum* 1987; **3**:481–8.
10. Sperling R, Larken J, Coblyn J et al. Methotrexate (MTX) decreases leukotriene B4 (LTB4) production in rheumatoid arthritis. 53rd Annual Meeting. American College of Rheumatology [abstract No. 14]. *Arthritis Rheum* 1989; **32**:S43.
11. Meyer FA, Yaron I, Mashiah V et al. Methotrexate inhibits proliferation but not interleukin 1 stimulated secretory activites of cultured human synovial fibroblasts. *J Rheumatol* 1993; **20**:238–42.
12. Scheven BAA, Van der Veen MJ, Damen CA et al. Effects of methotrexate on human osteoblasts in vitro: Modulation by 1,25-dihydroxyvitamin D3. *J Bone Miner Res* 1995; **10**:874–80.
13. Segal R, Yaron M, Tartakovsky B. Rescue of interleukin-1 activity by leucovorin following inhibition by methotrexate in a murine in vitro system. *Arthritis Rheum* 1990; **33**:1745–8.
14. Dooley MA, Pisetsky DS, Dawson DV et al. Soluble serum IL-2 receptor levels in refractory RA: trends during MTX therapy [abstract No. 22]. *Arthritis Rheum* 1991:34.
15. Crilly A, Madhok R, Murphy E et al. Serum IL-6 and soluble IL-2 receptor levels in rheumatoid patients receiving methotrexate [abstract No. 28]. *Clin Rheumatol* 1993 **12**:121.
16. Barrera P, Boerbooms AMT, Janssen EM et al. Circulating soluble tumour necrosis factor receptors, interleukin-2 receptors, tumor necrosis factor α, and interleukin-6 levels in rheumatoid arthritis. Longitudinal evaluation during methotrexate and azathioprine therapy. *Arthritis Rheum* 1993; **36**:1070–9.

17. Seitz M, Dewald B, Ceska M et al. Interleukin-8 in inflammatory rheumatic diseases; synovial fluid levels relation to rheumatoid factors, production by mononuclear cells, and effects of gold soldium thiomalate and methotrexate. *Rheumatol Int* 1992; **12**:159–64.
18. Bologna C, Edno L, Anaya JM, Canovas F et al. Methotrexate concentrations in synovial membrane and trabecular and cortical bone in rheumatoid arthritis patients. *Arthritis Rheum* 1994; **37**:1770–3.
19. Hansten PH, Horn J. Methotrexate and nonsteroidal anti-inflammatory drugs. *Drug Interact Newslett* 1986; **6**:41–3.
20. Shen DD, Azarnoff DL. Clinical pharmacokinetics of methotrexate. *Clin Pharmacokinet* 1978; **3**:1–13.
21. Kremer JM, Lee JK. The safety and efficacy of the use of methotrexate in long-term therapy for rheumatoid arthritis. *Arthritis Rheum* 1986; **29**:822–31.
22. Weinblatt ME, Trentham DE, Fraser PA et al. Long-term prospective trial of low-dose methotrexate in rheumatoid arthritis. *Arthritis Rheum* 1988; **31**:167–75.
23. Weinblatt ME. Toxicity of low dose methotrexate in rheumatoid arthritis. *J Rheumatol* 1985; **12**:35–9.
24. Dubin HV, Harrell ER. Liver disease associated with methotrexate treatment of psoriatic patients. *Arch Dermatol* 1970; **102**:498–503.
25. Shergy WJ, Polisson RP, Caldwell DS, Rice JR, Pisetsky DS, Allen NB. Methotrexate-associated hepatotoxicity: Retrospective analysis of 210 patients with rheumatoid arthritis. *Am J Med* 1988; **85**:771–4.
26. Kremer JM, Lee RG, Tolman KG. Liver histology in rheumatoid arthritis patients receiving long-term methotrexate therapy. A prospective study with baseline and sequential biopsy samples. *Arthritis Rheum* 1989; **32**: 121–7.
27. Kremer JM, Kaye GI, Kaye NW, Ishak KG, Axiotis CA. Light and electron microscopic analysis of sequential liver biopsy samples from rheumatoid arthritis patients receiving long-term methotrexate therapy. Followup over long treatment intervals and correlation with clinical and laboratory variables. *Arthritis Rheum* 1995; **38**:1194–203.
28. Weinblatt M, Walker AM, Funch D et al. Serious liver disease in methotrexate-treated RA patients [abstract]. *Arthritis Rheum* 1991; **34**:S49.
29. White-O'Keefe QF, Fye KH, Sack KD. Liver biopsy and methotrexate use: See no evil.... *Am J Gastroenterol* 1991; **70**:711–16.
30. Houtman PM, Stenger AME, Bruyn GAW, Mulder J, Dawson TM, Ryan PFJ. Methotrexate may affect certain T lymphocyte subsets in rheumatoid arthritis resulting in susceptility to *Pneumocystis carinii. J Rheum* 1994; **21**:1168–70.
31. Schnabel A, Burchardi C, Gross WL, Boerbooms AMT, Kerstens PJSM, Van Leophout JWA, Van de Putte L. Major infection during methotrexate treatment for rheumatoid arthritis. *Semin Arthritis Rheum* 1996; **25**:357–9.
32. Thompson RW, Craig FE, Banks PM, Sears DL, Myerson GE, Gulley ML. Epstein–Barr virus and lymphoproliferation in methotrexate-treated rheumatoid arthritis. *Mod Pathol* 1996; **9**:261–6.
33. Carpenter MT, West SG, Vogelgesang SA, Jones DEC. Postoperative joint infections in rheumatoid arthritis patients on methotrexate therapy. *Orthopedics* 1996; **19**:207–10.
34. St Clair EW, Rice JR, Synderman R. Pneumonitis complicating low-dose methotrexate therapy in rheumatoid arthritis. *Arch Int Med* 1985; **145**:2035–8.
35. Carroll GJ, Thomas R, Phatouros CC, Atchison MH, Leslie AL, Cook NJ, De Souza I. Incidence, prevalence and possible risk factors for pneumonitis in patients with rheumatoid arthritis receiving methotrexate. *J Rheum* 1994; **21**:51–4.
36. Beyeler C, Jordi B, Gerber NJ, Hof V. Pulmonary function in rheumatoid arthritis treated with low-dose methotrexate: A longitudinal study. *Br Rheum* 1996; **35**:446–52.
37. Lin WY, Kao CH, Wang SJ, Yeh SH. Lung toxicity of chemotherapeutic agents detected by TC-99 DTPA radioaerosol inhalation lung scintigraphy. *Neoplasma* 1995; **42**:133–5.
38. Carson CW, Cannon GW, Egger MJ et al. Pulmonary disease during the treatment of rheumatoid arthritis with low dose pulse methotrexate. *Semin Arthritis Rheum* 1987; **16**:186–95.
39. Hargreaves MR, Mowat AG, Benson MK. Acute pneumonitis associated with low dose methotrexate treatment for rheumatoid arthritis: report of 5 cases and review of published reports. *Thorax* 1992; **47**:628–33.
40. Meister B, Gassner I, Streif W, Dengg K, Fink FM. Methotrexate osteopathy in infants with tumours of the central nervous system. *Med Pediatr Oncol* 1994; **23**:493–6.
41. May KP, West SC, McDermott MT, Huffer WE. The effect of low-dose methotrexate on bone metabolism and histomorphometry in rats. *Arthritis Rheum* 1994; **37**:201–6.

42. Feldkamp M, Carey JC. Clinical teratology counselling and consultation case report: Low dose methotrexate exposure in the early weeks of pregnancy. *Teratology* 1993; **47**:533–9.
43. Morris LF, Harrod MJ, Menter MA, Silverman AK. Methotrexate and reproduction in men: Case report and recommendations. *J Am Acad Dermatol* 1993; **29**:913–16.
44. Kerr LD, Troy K, Isola L. Temporal association between the use of methotrexate and development of leukemia in 2 patients with rheumatoid arthritis. *J Rheum* 1995; **22**:2356–8.
45. Kamel OW, Van de Rijn M, Weiss LM et al. Reversible lymphomas associated with Epstein–Barr virus occurring during methotrexatae therapy for rheumatoid arthritis and dermatomyositis. *N Engl J Med* 1993; **328**:1317–21.
46. Wysocka K, Petrus B. Long-term treatment with imuran and methotrexate in rheumatoid condiutions. *Reumatologia* 1972; **10**:35–41.
47. Skinner MD, Schwartz RS. Immunosuppressive therapy. 1. *N Engl J Med* 1972; **287**:221–7.
48. Rodnan GP. Psoriatic arthritis. *J Am Med Assoc* 1973; **224**(5 Suppl):732–2.
49. Hoffmeister RT. Methotrexate therapy in rheumatoid arthritis: 15 years experience. *Am J Med* 1983; **75**:69–73.
50. Weinblatt ME, Coblyn JS, Fox DA et al. Efficacy of low-dose methotrexate in rheumatoid arthritis. *N Engl J Med* 1985; **312**:818–22.
51. Williams HJ, Willkens RF, Samuelson CO et al. Comparison of low-dose oral pulse methotrexate and placebo in the treatment of rheumatoid arthritis. A controlled clinical trial. *Arthritis Rheum* 1985; **28**:721–30.
52. Andersen PA, West SG, O'Dell JR et al. Weekly pulse methotrexate in rheumatoid arthritis. *Ann Intern Med* 1985; **103**:489–96.
53. Weinblatt ME, Maier AL. Longterm experience with low dose weekly methotrexate in rheumatoid arthritis. *J Rheum* 1990; **17**:33–8.
54. Felson DT, Anderson JJ, Meenan RF. The comparative efficacy and toxicity of second-line drugs in rheumatoid arthritis: Results of two meta-analyses. *Arthritis Rheum* 1990; **33**:1449–61.
55. Felson DT, Anderson JJ, Meenan RF. Use of short-term efficacy–toxicity tradeoffs to select second-line drugs in rheumatoid arthritis. A meta-analysis of published clinical trials. *Arthritis Rheum* 1992; **35**:1117–25.
56. Weinblatt ME, Kaplan H, Germain B et al. Methotrexate in rheumatoid arthritis. A five-year prospective multicenter study. *Arthritis Rheum* 1994; **10**:1492–7.
57. Tugwell P, Bombardier C, Buchanan WW et al. Methotrexate in rheumatoid arthritis. Impact on quality of life assessed by traditional standard-item and individualized patient preference health status questionnaires. *Arch Int Med* 1990; **150**:59–62.
58. Hanrahan PS, Scrivens GA, Russell AS. Prospective long-term follow-up of methotrexate therapy in rheumatoid arthritis: Toxicity, efficacy and radiological progression. *Br J Rheum* 1989; **28**:147–53.
59. Reykdal S, Steinsson K. Sigurjonsson K, Brekkan A. Methotrexate treatment of rheumatoid arthritis: effects on radiological progression. *Scand J Rheum* 1989; **18**:221–6.
60. Alarcon GS, Lopez-Mendez A, Walter J et al. Radiographic evidence of disease progression in methotrexate treated and nonmethotrexate disease modifying antirheumatic drug treated rheumatoid arthritis patients: a meta-analysis. *J Rheumatol* 1992; **19**:1868–73.
61. Lopez-Mendez A, Daniel WW, Reading JC, Ward JR, Alarcon GS. Radiographic assessment of disease progression in rheumatoid arthritis patients enrolled in the Cooperative Systematic Studies of the Rheumatic Diseases program randomized clinical trial of methotrexate, auranofin, or a combination of the two. *Arthritis Rheum* 1993; **36**:1364–9.
62. Rau R, Herborn G. Healing phenomena of erosive changes in rheumatoid arthritis patients undergoing disease-modifying antirheumatic drug therapy. *Arthritis Rheum* 1996; **30**:162–8.
63. Tugwell P, Pincus T, Yogum D et al. Combination therapy with cyclosporine and methotrexate in severe rheumatoid arthritis. *N Engl J Med* 1995; **333**:137–41.
64. Odell JR, Haire CE, Erikson N et al. Treatment of rheumatoid arthritis with methotrexate alone, sulfasalazine and hydroxychloroquine, or a combination of all three. *N Engl J Med* 1996; **334**:1287–91.
65. Healey LA, Wilke KR. Reforming the pyramid. A plan for treating rheumatoid arthritis in the 1990's. *Rheum Dis Clin North Am* 1989; **15**:615–19.
66. Fries JF. Re-evaluating the therapeutic approach to rheumatoid arthritis: The 'sawtooth' strategy. *J Rheum* 1990; **17**:12–15.
67. Van der Heide A, Jacobs JWG, Bijlsma JWJ et al. The effectiveness of early treatment with 'second-line' antirheumatic drugs. A randomized controlled trial. *Ann Int Med* 1996; **124**:699–707.
68. Heberden W. *Commentaries on the History and Cure of Diseases*, 1782:71.

5

What is the likely role of monoclonal antibody therapy in the treatment of rheumatoid arthritis?

Ernest HS Choy, Gabrielle H Kingsley and Gabriel S Panayi

INTRODUCTION

The development of monoclonal antibody (mAb) was greeted with optimism as 'the golden bullet' that would revolutionize tumour therapy and the treatment of chronic inflammatory diseases such as rheumatoid arthritis (RA). Controversies arose, as data from initial clinical trials were disappointing. The protagonists of mAb maintain that this is a complex biological treatment requiring much more development, whilst the opponents argue that the whole hypothesis on which mAb therapy is based is flawed. This review uses the results of trials of anti-tumour necrosis factor-α (TNFα) and anti-T-cell mAb therapy to explore this controversy.

MONOCLONAL ANTIBODIES

Antibodies are immunoglobulin (Ig) molecules; each is made up of a variable region (Fab), which binds antigen, and a constant region (Fc). The latter, depending on the class and subclass of the Fc, may bind to Fc receptors or fix complement. Depending on the objective of therapy, an antigen-specific Fab can be joined to a selected Ig isotype to mediate different functions, such as antibody-dependent cytotoxicity or complement-mediated cytolysis.

Monoclonal antibodies directed against human targets are usually produced in mice. One of the major problems associated with the use of murine mAb in humans is the development of a human anti-mouse (HAMA) response. There are two main types of anti-globulin response: anti-isotypic and anti-idiotypic. The former is usually directed against the Fc region of the mAb, whereas the latter binds to the Fab. HAMA responses lead to two main drawbacks: first, retreatment may result in anaphylaxis and, second, retreatments may be less effective therapeutically. Advances in molecular biology have helped to produce engineered antibodies with the aim of reducing their antigenicity.[1] These are of two types: a chimaeric mAb is a construct of the murine antibody Fab and the human immunoglobulin Fc, whereas a humanized mAb is a construct in which the whole of the murine mAb, apart from the complementarity-determining regions which bind antigen, has been replaced by human Ig proteins (Figure 5.1).

HYPOTHESIS: PATHOGENESIS OF RHEUMATOID ARTHRITIS

One of the controversies in the pathogensis of RA concerns the role of T cells and cytokines in the perpetuation of chronic disease.[2] In general, most researchers agree that RA is initiated by an arthritogenic peptide presented by the major histocompatibility class II molecule,

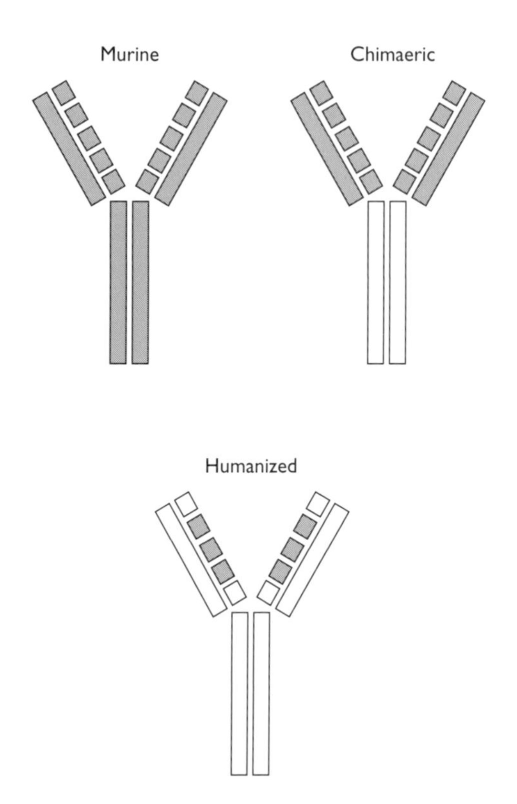

Figure 5.1 Different types of monoclonal antibody. Shaded and clear areas indicate murine and human sequences, respectively.

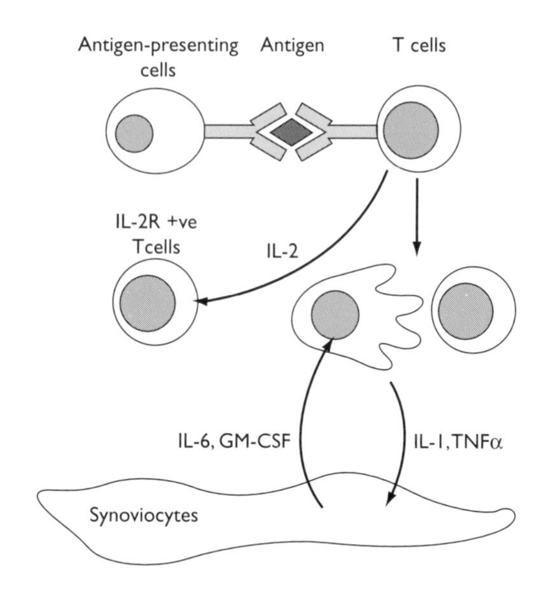

Figure 5.2 Cytokine network in rheumatoid arthritis. IFNγ, interferon γ; IL, interleukin; TNFα, tumour necrosis factor α; GM-CSF, granulocyte–monocyte colony stimulating factor.

HLA-DR4/DR1, of antigen-presenting cells to CD4+ T cells[3] (Figure 5.2). Activated CD4+ T cells produce the lymphokines, interleukin (IL)-2 and interferon γ (IFNγ), which initiate the inflammatory cascade. Both IFNγ and activated CD4+ T cells, the latter through direct contact, stimulate monocytes and synoviocytes to produce IL-1 and TNFα.[4] These activate other mesenchymal cells to produce other cytokines such as IL-6 and granulocyte–monocyte colony stimulating factor (GM-CSF). Furthermore, IL-1 and TNFα stimulate the production of matrix metalloproteinases which are the enzymes ultimately responsible for joint damage in RA.[5,6]

However, IL-2 and IFNγ are present only in very small amounts in rheumatoid synovia, the predominant cytokines being monokines such as TNFα and IL-1. Therefore, some researchers have argued that chronic established RA is perpetuated by a positive feedback loop between cytokines which include IL-1, TNFα, IL-6 and GM-CSF.[2] Data from the use of mAbs for the therapy of RA may provide interesting opportunities to investigate these competing hypotheses.

OVERVIEW OF MONOCLONAL ANTIBODY THERAPY IN RHEUMATOID ARTHRITIS WITH RELEVANCE TO PATHOGENESIS

The specificity of mAbs makes them unique for the treatment of autoimmune diseases. In the past, most therapies were nonspecific immunosuppressants, but mAbs allow the targeting of a specific mediator or cell involved in inflammation. Therefore, clinical trials using mAbs may offer new insights into the pathogenesis of autoimmune diseases.

Anti-TNFα monoclonal antibody in rheumatoid arthritis

Both chimaeric and humanized anti-TNFα mAbs have been used. Their development was based on in vitro and in vivo evidence that TNFα has an important role in the pathogenesis of RA.[7] TNFα is a very potent proinflammatory cytokine produced by monocytes/macrophages and synoviocytes in RA. It can be detected in the blood and synovial joints of patients with RA.[8,9] Mice transgenic for human TNFα produce high levels of TNFα constitutively and develop a spontaneous inflammatory, destructive polyarthritis resembling RA.[10] Furthermore, in collagen-induced arthritis, disease can be treated effectively by anti-TNFα mAb.[11] These in vivo data are supported by in vitro experiments in which TNFα induced the production of other proinflammatory cytokines such as IL-1, IL-6 and GM-CSF.[12-14]

High-dose anti-TNFα mAb (10 mg/kg) produced dramatic anti-inflammatory effects in placebo-controlled trials.[15,16] Clinical improvement showed a clear dose response; 0.1 mg/kg was ineffective but 10 mg/kg produced disease amelioration within 1 week that peaked after 2 weeks. There were parallel decreases in acute phase reactants such as the erythrocyte sedimentation rate and C-reactive protein level; this may have been due to a reduction in circulating IL-6. This observation is of interest, as IL-6 is thought to be the inducer of the production of acute phase reactants from hepatocytes and its production is induced by TNFα.[13] Moreover, after treatment there was an approximately 25% reduction in levels of serum stromelysin and urine bone markers such as pyridinoline and deoxypyridinoline cross-links, suggesting that bone and cartilage destruction was also reduced.[17] These data confirm the hypothesis that TNFα is an important inducer of IL-6 and stromelysin production in RA. However, treatment with anti-TNFα mAb did not produce sustained clinical improvement, since, depending on the dose of mAb given, the duration of clinical improvement lasted only between 2–6 weeks. Repeated treatments were necessary in order to maintain clinical improvement,[18,19] suggesting that, even at high doses of anti-TNFα mAb, it is impossible to switch off disease and so produce prolonged remission. These data imply that, in established RA disease, there is continuous immune activation. This is supported by the high levels of the T cell immunoreactants sIL-2R and sCD4, which persisted in the serum of patients who had shown a good clinical and laboratory response with anti-TNFα mAb.[20] This implies that the CD4+ lymphocyte activation continues in chronic established RA, despite anti-TNFα mAb therapy.

One of the surprising findings in these clinical trials was the development of anti-double-stranded DNA and anti-phospholipid antibodies in some patients after treatment with anti-TNFα mAbs.[18,19] The mechanism of this is unknown but may be due to elevation in the IL-10 level. There is also concern that prolonged TNFα blockade may lead to the development of lymphoproliferative diseases and malignancies, because of the role of TNFα in tumour immunosurveillance. Clearly, if continuous TNFα blockade is necessary to control RA, the risk of these side-effects must be assessed in long-term clinical trials.

Anti-T-cell monoclonal antibody

T cells are the initiators of the cell-mediated immune response and therefore are attractive targets for immunotherapy. Initially, the aim of mAb treatment was to deplete T cells. This approach is supported by the success of total lymphoid irradiation, thoracic duct drainage and lymphocytopheresis. A number of humanized and chimaeric mAbs that deplete T cells have been used in RA; these include Campath-1H (humanized anti-CDw52 mAb), anti-CD7, CD5-plus (murine anti-CD5 mAb conjugated to ricin), and cM-T412 (chimaeric anti-CD4 mAb). To date, the results of depleting anti-T-cell mAbs have been disappointing,[21–23] but they have shared one important common feature. Lymphopenia induced by these mAbs was protracted, and therefore the risk of long-term immunosuppression limits the dose of treatment which can be given. We will highlight this problem using the example of Campath-1H and cM-T412.

Campath-1H is a humanized mAb that targets the pan-T-cell antigen CDw52. It leads to complement-mediated lysis of the target cell and treatment leads to profound lymphopenia. In open clinical trials,[24–26] it improved disease, although this improvement did not correlate with the degree of lymphopenia. Indeed, disease often relapsed, despite profound lymphopenia. However, when the synovia were examined in these patients, CD4 lymphocytes were still present in large numbers. This may be due to failure of Campath-1H to reach the joint, or to the fact that synovial T cells are more resistant to lysis at the dosage given. The failure to deplete synovial lymphocytes by anti-T-cell mAbs was also found with other antibodies, including cM-T412.

The chimaeric anti-CD4 mAb, cM-T412 (Centocor), also led to significant depletion of peripheral blood CD4 cells after a single 50-mg injection. After repeated treatments (50 mg daily for 5 days), there was a severe and prolonged peripheral blood CD4 lymphopenia exacerbated by concomitant therapy with methotrexate or a corticosteroid.[27,28] Interestingly, the decrease in synovial fluid CD4 lymphocyte number was much less than that found in the peripheral blood.[28] The clinical response was variable, but correlated with the percentage of synovial fluid CD4 lymphocytes that were coated with cM-T412. The concentration of cM-T412 found in the joint was low, implying that higher doses would be necessary for a consistent therapeutic effect. However, the dosage was limited by the profound peripheral blood CD4 lymphopenia. Because of the CD4 lymphopenia, the development of depleting anti-CD4 mAbs has ceased. Use of nondepleting anti-CD4 mAbs may circumvent this impasse; a number of these are being currently tested in RA.

The continued presence of synovial CD4+ lymphocytes in the joints of patients treated with anti-T-cell mAbs probably explains the low incidence of opportunistic infections. However, these have been seen in patients treated with high doses of Campath-1H[29] and a combination of anti-CD4 mAbs and methotrexate.[27] Another possible limiting factor for anti-T-cell therapy may be the development of cytokine release syndrome. This is characterized by pyrexia, chills, rigor and hypotension. The severity of the cytokine release syndrome produced varies greatly amongst anti-T-cell mAbs. Campath-1H induced a severe cytokine release syndrome in all patients, but cM-T412 led to a mild reaction in a small number of patients.

Because of these results, depleting anti-T-cell therapies have been abandoned, but nondepleting anti-T-cell mAbs may be the next step. In animal models of arthritis, such as streptococcal cell wall arthritis and collagen-induced arthritis, it has been shown that treatment with nondepleting anti-CD4 mAbs could lead to long-term disease improvement[30,31] by the induction of immunological tolerance. In these models, an inflammatory arthritis similar to RA develops after injection with streptococcal cell walls or immunization with type II collagen. If nondepleting anti-CD4 mAbs are given at the time of disease induction, the treated animals do not develop arthritis. Furthermore, if the animals are reinjected again 6 weeks later, they are resistant to arthritis reinduction without further treatment with anti-CD4 mAbs. Recent data in RA with the use of primatized and humanized nondepleting anti-CD4 mAbs led to significant disease improvement, but whether these can induce immunological tolerance remains to be assessed in long-term studies.

CONTROVERSY

In order to assess the value of a potential therapy for RA accurately, one must define the objectives of treatment. Despite treatment with disease-modifying antirheumatic drugs (DMARDs), the long-term outcome of RA remains poor.[32] The main concern with DMARDs is that few patients can continue with treatment after 5 years,[33] because of side-effects and lack of efficacy. The ideal treatment of RA is one that is safe and produces sustained disease remission after a brief course of treatment. Short of this, new treatments must suppress inflammation and retard radiological damage. If repeated treatments are necessary, then they must be safe and economical to use in the long term.

Cost

Monoclonal antibodies are expensive, in that large quantities are often necessary to control disease and the cost of production is high. In the case of anti-TNFα mAb, 10 mg/kg is necessary to improve disease and treatments need to be repeated every 4–8 weeks. As the sole treatment for RA, anti-TNFα therapy would clearly be very expensive. However, anti-TNFα mAb could be used in conjunction with conventional DMARDs, such as methotrexate, in three situations. First, in acute disease flares, it should be efficacious and will be particularly useful in patients who are steroid resistant. Second, as most DMARDs have a slow onset of action, anti-TNFα mAb given at the initiation of DMARD treatment will control disease more rapidly, and this may be especially relevant in early RA. Third, it can be used in combination with DMARDs when disease control with the latter is suboptimal, although there is the possible risk of increased immunosuppression. There is also the additional cost of frequent repeated intravenous infusion and monitoring for infusion-related toxicity. If a short course of mAb could produce sustained disease improvement, then these cost constraints would disappear and it would be feasible for it to be used in routine clinical practice. On the positive side, although the cost of mAb is much higher than that of current DMARDs, the latter require regular blood tests to monitor side-effects; such monitoring is extremely expensive.[34,35] Comer et al found that the cost of monitoring was approximately £270/year in the UK,[34] while Prashker et al found that the cost of treatment with DMARDs, including monitoring, ranged from $552/year to $1606/year in the USA.[35] Therefore, the cost of mAb may be comparable to that of conventional DMARDs, if a short course of treatment produced prolonged benefit without the requirement for blood tests.

Long-term efficacy/toxicity

If repeated mAb treatments are necessary to control disease activity with mAb such as anti-TNFα, then the development of HAMA becomes likely, despite the fact that chimaerization and humanization of mAbs have reduced antibody antigenicity. Studies with chimaeric and humanized antibodies have shown that, with repeated administration, many patients will develop anti-antibody responses. Two strategies could circumvent this problem: first, is the co-administration of the mAb with an anti-CD4 mAb to induce tolerance to the mouse protein component of the mAb. This possibility needs to be formally tested in clinical trials. Second, is the avoidance of mAb by the use, when these are available, of alternative strategies, such as the infusion of a soluble receptor–human Ig construct.

Monoclonal antibodies bind to their targets with high affinity and, when they are directed against targets such as lymphocytes and cytokines, they could result in significant immunosuppression. Furthermore, lymphocytes and cytokines, in particular TNFα, are involved in tumour surveillance. Prolonged suppression may lead to increased incidence of tumours, especially leukaemias and lymphomas.

Clinical practice

At present, mAbs are administered as intravenous infusions. Clearly, medical supervision is required, and this increases the cost of treatment. Furthermore, if frequent and regular treatments are required, then they may be impractical for many rheumatology departments. However, providing the dose of antibody required for treatment is small, antibody could be administered either subcutaneously or intramuscularly, although such routes of administration could theoretically increase the likelihood of the development of anti-globulin antibodies.

CONCLUSIONS

The limitation of DMARDs leaves a significant proportion of RA patients without effective treatment. Any addition to the current treatments would be welcomed if it is efficacious, nontoxic and practical for clinical use. Monoclonal antibodies offer the opportunity of developing therapies that are short in duration, produce prolonged disease remission, and are without significant toxicity.

ACKNOWLEDGMENTS

The Rheumatology Unit is supported by grants from the Arthritis and Rheumatism Council for Great Britain. The studies utilizing cM-T412 and CDP571 were sponsored by Centocor Ltd and Celltech Therapeutics Ltd, respectively.

REFERENCES

1. Winter G, Milstein C. Man-made antibodies. *Nature* 1991; **349**:293–9.
2. Firestein GS, Zvaifler NJ. How important are T cells in chronic rheumatoid synovitis? *Arthritis Rheum* 1990; **33**:768–73.
3. Panayi GS, Lanchbury JS, Kingsley GH. The importance of the T cell in inititiating and maintaining the chronic synovitis of rheumatoid arthritis. *Arthritis Rheum* 1992; **35**:729–35.
4. Isler P, Vey E, Zhang JH, Dayer JM. Cell surface glycoproteins expressed on activated human T cells induce production of interleukin-1 beta by monocytic cells: a possible role of CD69. *Eur Cytokine Network* 1993; **4**:15–23.
5. MacNaul KL, Chartrain N, Lark M, Tocci MJ, Hutchinson NI. Discoordinate expression of stromelysin, collagenase, and tissue inhibitor of metalloproteinases-1 in rheumatoid human synovial fibroblasts. Synergistic effects of interleukin-1 and tumor necrosis factor-alpha on stromelysin expression. *J Biol Chem* 1990; **265**:17 238–45.
6. Shingu M, Nagai Y, Isayama T, Naono T, Nobunaga M. The effects of cytokines on metalloproteinase inhibitors (TIMP) and collagenase production by human chondrocytes and TIMP production by synovial cells and endothelial cells. *Clin Exp Immunol* 1993; **94**:145–9.
7. Brennan FM, Maini RN, Feldmann M. TNF alpha – a pivotal role in rheumatoid arthritis? *Br J Rheumatol* 1992; **31**:293–8.
8. Chu CQ, Field M, Allard S, Abney E, Feldmann M, Maini RM. Detection of cytokines at the cartilage/pannus junction in patients with rheumatoid arthritis: implications for the role of cytokines in cartilage destruction and repair. *Br J Rheumatol* 1992; **31**:653–61.
9. Barrera P, Boerbooms AM, Janssen EM et al. Circulating soluble tumor necrosis factor receptors, interleukin-2 receptors, tumor necrosis factor alpha, and interleukin-6 levels in rheumatoid arthritis. Longitudinal evaluation during methotrexate and azathioprine therapy *Arthritis Rheum* 1993; **36**:1070–9.
10. Keffer J, Probert L, Cazlaris H et al. Transgenic mice expressing human tumour necrosis factor: a predictive genetic model of arthritis. *EMBO J* 1991; **10**:4025–31.
11. Williams RO, Feldmann M, Maini RN. Anti-tumor necrosis factor ameliorates joint disease in murine collagen-induced arthritis. *Proc Natl Acad Sci USA* 1992; **89**:9784–8.
12. Brannan FM, Chantry D, Jackson A, Maini RN, Feldmann M. Inhibitory effect of TNFα antibodies on synovial cell interleukin-1 production in rheumatoid arthritis. *Lancet* 1989; **ii**:244–7.
13. Akira S, Hirano T, Taga T, Kishimoto T. Biology of multifunctional cytokines: IL6 and related molecules (IL1 and TNF). *FASEB J* 1990; **4**:2860–7.
14. Alvaro Gracia JM, Zvaifler NJ, Firestein GS. Cytokines in chronic inflammatory arthritis. V. Mutual antagonism between interferon-gamma and tumor necrosis factor-alpha on HLA-DR expression, proliferation, collagenase production, and granulocyte macrophage colony-stimulating factor production by rheumatoid arthritis synoviocytes. *J Clin Invest* 1990; **86**:1790–8.
15. Rankin EC, Choy EH, Kassimos D et al. The therapeutic effects of an engineered human anti-tumour necrosis factor alpha antibody (CDP571) in rheumatoid arthritis. *Br J Rheumatol* 1995; **34**:334–42.

16. Elliott MJ, Maini RN, Feldmann M et al. Randomised double-blind comparison of chimeric monoclonal antibody to tumour necrosis factor α (cA2) versus placebo in rheumatoid arthritis. *Lancet* 1994; **344**:1105–10.
17. Choy EHS, Kassimos D, Kingsley GH et al. The effect of an engineered human anti-tumour necrosis factor alpha (TNFα) antibody (Ab) on interleukin-6 (IL-6) and bone markers in rheumatoid arthritis (RA) patients. *Arthritis Rheum* 1995; **38** (Suppl):S185.
18. Elliott MJ, Maini RN, Feldmann M et al. Repeated therapy with monoclonal antibody to tumour necrosis factor α (cA2) in patients with rheumatoid arthritis. *Lancet* 1994; **344**:1125–7.
19. Rankin ECC, Choy EHS, Sopwith M et al. Repeated doses of 10 mg/kg of an engineered human anti-TNFα antibody, CDP571, in RA patients are safe and effective. *Arthritis Rheum* 1995; **38** (Suppl):S185
20. Choy EHS, Rankin ECC, Kassimos D et al. Engineered human anti-tumour necrosis factor alpha (TNFα) antibody (Ab) reduces serum interleukin-6 (IL-6) and urine bone markers but has no effect on soluble CD4 (sCD4) and soluble interleukin-2 receptor (sIL2R) in rheumatoid arthritis (RA). *Br J Rheumatol* 1996; **35** (Suppl):172
21. Choy EHS, Chikanza IC, Kingsley GH, Corrigall V, Panayi GS. Treatment of rheumatoid arthritis with single dose or weekly pulses of chimaeric anti-CD4 monoclonal antibody. *Scand J Immunol* 1992; **36**:291–8.
22. Moreland LW, Bucy RP, Tilden A et al. Use of a chimeric monoclonal anti-CD4 antibody in patients with refractory rheumatoid arthritis. *Arthritis Rheum* 1993; **36**:307–18.
23. van der Lubbe PA, Dijkmans BA, Markusse HM, Nassander U, Breedveld FC. A randomized, double-blind, placebo-controlled study of CD4 monoclonal antibody therapy in early rheumatoid arthritis. *Arthritis Rheum* 1995; **38**(8): 1097–106.
24. Isaacs JD, Watts RA, Hazelman BL et al. Humanised monoclonal antibody therapy for rheumatoid arthritis. *Lancet* 1992; **340**:748–52.
25. Matteson EL, Yocum DE, St Clair EW et al. Treatment of active refractory rheumatoid arthritis with humanized monoclonal antibody CAMPATH-1H administered by daily subcutaneous injection. *Arthritis Rheum* 1995; **38**:1187–93.
26. Isaacs JD, Manna VK, Rapson N et al. Campath-1H in rheumatoid arthritis – an intravenous dose-ranging study. *Br J Rheumatol* 1996; **35**:231–40.
27. Moreland LW, Pratt PW, Bucy RP, Jackson BS, Feldman JW, Koopman WJ. Treatment of refractory rheumatoid arthritis with chimaeric anti-CD4 antibody. Long-term follow up of CD4+ T cell counts. *Arthritis Rheum* 1994; **37**:834–8.
28. Choy EH, Pitzalis C, Cauli A et al. Percentage of anti-CD4 monoclonal antibody-coated lymphocytes in the rheumatoid joint is associated with clinical improvement. Implications for the development of immunotherapeutic dosing regimens. *Arthritis Rheum* 1996; **39**:52–6.
29. Poynton CH, Mort D, Maughan TS. Adverse reactions to Campath-1H monoclonal antibody. *Lancet* 1993; **341**:1037.
30. Van den Broek MF, Van de Langerijt LG, Van Bruggen MC, Billingham ME, Van den Berg WB. Treatment of rats with monoclonal anti-CD4 induces long-term resistance to streptococcal cell wall-induced arthritis. *Eur J Immunol* 1992; **22**:57–61.
31. Billingham ME, Hicks C, Carney S. Monoclonal antibodies and arthritis. *Agents Action* 1990; **29**:77–87.
32. Scott DL, Symmons DP, Coulton BL, Popert AJ. Long-term outcome of treating rheumatoid arthritis: results after 20 years. *Lancet* 1987; **1**:1108–11.
33. Wijnands MJ, van't Hof MA, van Leeuwen MA, van Rijswijk MH, van de Putte LB, van Riel PL. Long-term second-line treatment: a prospective drug survival study. *Br J Rheumatol* 1992; **31**:253–8.
34. Comer M, Scott DL, Doyle DV, Huskisson EC, Hopkins A. Are slow-acting anti-rheumatic drugs monitored too often? An audit of current clinical practice. *Br J Rheumatol* 1995; **34**:966–70.
35. Prashker MJ, Meenan RF. The total costs of drug therapy for rheumatoid arthritis. A model based on costs of drug, monitoring, and toxicity. *Arthritis Rheum* 1995; **38**:318–25.

6

Managing chronic pain – can rheumatologists do it better?

Michael Shipley

Pain is the commonest complaint of patients who visit a rheumatologist. It varies in severity, duration and impact on the individual's life. Pain is sometimes easy to understand and, indeed, protective, for example, after an accident or when a joint is swollen and inflamed, or when a disc has prolapsed and is causing nerve root irritation. The person in pain may need to have the cause explained by a skilled diagnostician, but once the cause is understood the pain can be more readily coped with, particularly if it is expected to get better. The plethora of analgesic and anti-inflammatory agents, of newer pain-relieving techniques and of physical methods all help, when used appropriately. In some situations, however, the cause of the pain is less clear, not only to the individual but also to the medical advisor. When such pain persists, it brings with it additional changes in perception and in behaviour, and the resultant disability may worsen. Managing chronic pain, which arises from mainly non-life-threatening causes, is one of the greatest challenges that rheumatologists face. Appropriate early management, adequate pain control, and prevention of persistent inflammation and consequent damage can all help. Addressing the impact of pain on the individual in his or her broader social and psychological context will also contribute to preventing chronic pain syndromes.

Those treating pain require an understanding not just of the newer neurophysiological evidence about the structure and plasticity of the nervous system, but also of the psychological, social, and cultural aspects of pain. Pain is a personal and subjective experience. It is influenced by the way in which the peripheral and central nervous systems are changed by the initial cause and by subsequent events. The impact of pain can be influenced by cultural learning and attitudes to pain, by the particular meaning of the situation to the individual, by changes in attention to the pain and by other psychological variables. It can no longer be thought of in the traditional Cartesian dualistic model, by which an unchangeable line carries information to the brain, where it is then interpreted as pain.

Understanding the acquired or learned attitude of the individual towards their pain requires time and patience. It is no longer acceptable for the clinician to assume that 'unexplained' pain, that is pain without an obvious pathophysiological cause, is 'all in the mind' or the result of a disordered personality. There is now a mass of evidence that begins to explain the variation in pain severity in, for example, osteoarthritis or rheumatoid arthritis – pain that appears, to a greater or lesser extent, to be independent of the clearly demonstrable joint pathology. In this context it becomes easier for the clinician to understand and accept chronic pain syndromes, of which the physical cause is more difficult to detect. It is helpful to think of all chronic painful problems as being the result of both physical and psychological changes, even though the balance between the physical and the psychological will vary considerably between individuals, and in the same individual at different times.

NEUROPHYSIOLOGY OF PAIN

At this point some comments on newer aspects of the neurophysiology of pain may be appropriate. The gate control theory of pain[1] demonstrated that pain had only rarely a one-to-one relationship to the stimulus. This theory was a major conceptual leap to understanding pain perception as a complex, multifaceted phenomenon. Research into the gate control theory has clarified the plasticity of the central nervous system (CNS), the control through chemical mediators from normal peripheral neurological activity in the CNS, and the paramount importance of the spinal cord and brain in the handling of information, modulating it upwards or downwards in different circumstances, sometimes to beneficial effect but at other times with disastrous results. This phenomenon is called neuroplasticity. With the demonstration that permanent or long-lasting changes can be induced in the peripheral and central pain pathways, it became possible to understand, in broad terms, how apparently trivial initiating factors might lead to chronic pain. The concept that the brain can control the spinal cord, at both conscious and unconscious levels, encourages the open mind to believe that past experience and psychological and social factors can also affect pain perception. The assumption that the problem is either physical or psychological makes no sense in clinical practice. Patients and the community at large are all too often happy to believe, nonetheless, that there must be a physical cause, which, if only found and treated, would cure the chronic pain syndrome. The psychosocial factors may be too difficult to accept at face value and yet play an important role in most individuals. This mistaken belief is the cause of many inappropriate referrals and much overinvestigation. The patient with chronic pain may be difficult to manage and the cause of their pain difficult to understand, but, if clinicians accept the complexity of the situation and reduce their tendency to blame the patient for being difficult, interventions can be devised that will help. Clinicians can no longer retreat into the safe preserve of pathophysiological causation in which we have all been trained. The danger remains that clinicians may wash their hands of the problem, because no treatable cause has been found. Worst of all, the unresolved problem may be passed back, with a shrug of the shoulders, to the unprepared patient to deal with themselves. Much can be done for the patient suffering with chronic pain and the best setting for achieving this is usually a multiskilled pain clinic.

Individuals extract information from the mass of stimuli which affect them by (1) the ability of peripheral neurons to transmit the information, and (2) the ability of the dorsal horn and medulla to process it. A complex series of different conditions determines whether pain is perceived and, if it is, the quality of that pain.[2] The plentiful dorsal horn cells which have a wide dynamic range and which respond to low- and high-intensity peripheral stimuli are more likely to be responsible for the conscious appreciation of pain than are those nociceptive cells which respond to damaging and intense peripheral stimuli. At least some of these dorsal horn cells receive inputs, not from well defined and localized anatomical areas, but from a whole limb. This is a mechanism whereby initially localized pain can become more widespread.

Wall has proposed what he calls the 'reality/virtual reality' concept of pain.[3] This advances the concept of pain well beyond the earlier models. He suggests that two alternative pain mechanisms exist. In the 'reality' system there is no conscious perception. Appropriate behaviour is given the highest priority, according to an in-built repertoire, which can be modified by learning and experience. This system is in action in the pain/withdrawal reflex or the so-called emergency anaesthesia phenomenon. Wall also suggests that the reality system assigns pain a lower priority in the placebo response, because of a reduced expectation of pain; pain becomes effectively inappropriate. By contrast, in the 'virtual reality' system there is continuous observation and reassessment of sensory inputs 'as modified by a possible repertoire of alternative behaviours which would remove the stimulus. The operation of this circuit is conscious and is in action during perceived pain'. Wall cites two key observations in support of his theory.

First, experimental local anaesthetic blockade of the normal flow of relatively minor signals from a limb result in the phantom limb phenomenon. In the anaesthetic area it is not an imitation of the real limb but is exaggerated. The sensory input no longer fits a recognized repertoire, so the system creates its own virtual reality. In the experimental model, the subject can abolish the phantom limb by looking at or touching the anaesthetized limb. After amputation, this means of checking is not available and the phantom limb persists. Most readers have experienced the sensation of a swollen lip after a dental anaesthetic, although no swelling is apparent. Presumably the patient with severe carpal tunnel syndrome who complains of swollen fingers, even knowing they are not, is experiencing the same phenomenon.

Second, recordings are made from first order central cells receiving input from the skin. These cells normally fulfil all of the criteria for classical Cartesian transmission; they are reliable, predictable and anatomical. Monkeys are trained to discriminate and respond to stimuli and are rewarded when they respond appropriately. They are also given a warning that the stimulus is about to be applied. Once the animals are fully trained, a small number of the cells tested produce a brief burst of activity after the warning but before the stimulus has been applied. That is, the brain can be trained to create a virtual input which is in some ways identical to that produced by the stimulus itself.

Chronic pain syndromes may be virtual reality but nonetheless real for the person concerned. As Wall says of the virtual reality system, the person constantly 'observes and reassesses'. This becomes part of the problem, with excessive introspection and focus adding to the individual's distress. Like all clinicians, rheumatologists dealing with chronic pain must keep abreast of modern pain theory if they are to treat it appropriately.

PSYCHOLOGICAL ASPECTS OF PAIN

There is an extensive literature on psychological and emotional aspects of pain. The variety of types of pain is as complex as the language of pain. It is not that adequate words do not exist, rather that they are not part of the normal scientific vocabulary and may sound rather foolish. Anyone who has tried to describe pain will recognize this. When faced with a list of the most commonly used words, however, individuals will use them surprisingly consistently. This has been formalized in the studies which led to the creation of the McGill Pain Questionnaire (MPQ).[4] The MPQ takes the measurement of pain beyond the one-dimensional assumptions that are implicit in the visual analogue scale or in a pain score. It is not as easy to administer, but gives a better measure of the person's pain experience. It has been shown to be valid, reliable, consistent, and useful. Although the MPQ is more suited to the research setting than to the busy clinic, its messages are important for clinicians listening to and trying to understand patients as they struggle with words to describe their pain. Offering them a list may be a helpful prompt, because they are often very aware of the difficulties that their apparently melodramatic descriptions create in the observer. Allowing them to know that others use such words is, in practice, to give them permission to use the most appropriate words for themselves. Giving someone the time and means to talk about their chronic pain is a key to gaining their confidence and obtaining insight into their experience of it and, thereby, enables them to be treated effectively.

Pain behaviour is thought to be anomalous only when there is a significant mismatch between its reported severity and the observed physical disease. Experience and behaviour are usually correlated, but never completely so. Stoicism at one extreme or exaggeration to gain sympathy and attention at the other may lead the clinician to assess the level of subjective pain inaccurately, and usually to underestimate it. When there is a perceived discrepancy between the patient's verbal complaint of pain and nonverbal pain behaviour, the clinician usually deals with their personal dilemma by disregarding the patient's self-report.[5] This is a trap which a clinician must consciously and constantly avoid.

The aim of a behavioural approach to chronic pain is to treat excess disability and expressed suffering. The problem is how to define this excess disability and suffering accurately. It is important to encourage the patient but not to push them too far. Pain behaviour can be measured and may fall into recognizable patterns, but, alone, it cannot be assumed to indicate the level of pain.[6] A patient's pain behaviour may be an effective way of coping with pain and disability. It is only when the behaviour becomes ineffective that it is detrimental, yet it is extremely difficult to judge when this change from help to hindrance has occurred. This type of management requires judgments and skills in which a physician is usually inadequately trained. Rheumatologists must broaden their personal repertoire of skills and those of their team so that they increase the likelihood of getting these judgments right.

THE PLACEBO RESPONSE

Wall defines placebo as someone telling another what they expect and want to hear rather than the truth.[7] The importance of proving that a drug is more effective than a placebo is the basis of the double-blind placebo-controlled trial. Yet, in most studies, the 'placebo' treatment has effects too, producing both benefits and side-effects. These may not be as great as with the 'real' drug, but effects there are. Some participants actually prefer the placebo. In a study of analgesics of differing strengths vs placebo, the strength of the placebo effect was related to the strength of the analgesic with which it was being compared.[8] The power of the placebo appears to be dependent upon the expectation of the recipient. When a placebo is preceded by an analgesic, the effect of the placebo is increased. These observations demonstrate the power of impression and expectation. They should not be dismissed, nor used covertly lest the lie be discovered and the beneficial effect lost. Part of most consultations is just such a therapeutic act. The patient leaves the room expressing gratitude and feeling better, although 'all' that has been done is that the complaint has been listened to, paid due attention and given an adequate explanation. Suddenly the pain is less important, the fear less troublesome, and the patient reassured. The value of a consultation lies in a creative balance of different therapeutic interventions. A deeper understanding of the placebo effect will improve its more effective use. If, as Wall suggests, pain is felt only when it is deemed appropriate, is it possible to modify the individual's understanding of what is appropriate during the therapeutic relief of pain?

PAIN IN OSTEOARTHRITIS

Pain is the main problem for most people with osteoarthritis (OA). It is predominantly use-related, but around 50% of patients experience night pain and/or pain at rest. The mechanisms which cause the pain are poorly understood. Its perceived severity is dependent on age and the site of the affected joint and on the severity of radiological changes, but it is only partly explained by these factors. Anxiety and depression are important,[9] so it is logical that these be addressed in treatment.

OA is not a simple wear-and-tear phenomenon, but a final common pathway of degradation and repair processes. Even in severe OA a minority of articular chondrocytes remain able to synthesize matrix components. Repair is theoretically possible, and has been observed in some people. Disease-modifying agents for OA are still in the development stage. Simple analgesic agents, used when needed, help most people with OA to manage their pain and make life tolerable. Although nonsteroidal anti-inflammatory drugs (NSAIDs) are used widely, their high level of side-effects, especially in the elderly, is a disadvantage. Some NSAIDs may accelerate the destructive process in the joint by a direct detrimental effect on the chondrocyte,[10] others may be protective and, thus, more appropriate for use when simple or compound analgesics fail. Other therapeutic strategies combining exercise, education, weight loss, and the reduction of anxiety and depression all need to be considered, and help some individuals. The value of group working and shared experience is not adequately appreciated by doctors or physiotherapists. Salvage surgery is highly successful, but reflects the failure of rheumatologists and others to prevent pain and disability by preventing long-term joint damage in OA.

PAIN IN RHEUMATOID ARTHRITIS

Control of pain is one of the main demands of persons with rheumatoid arthritis (RA) and is generally underestimated by rheumatologists.[11] The inflamed joint is painful because of a complex series of changes which modify neuronal processing. Joint pain is normally produced only by extreme twisting or pressure. By contrast, however, resting pain is a feature of inflamed joints. Such joints may also be painful with only gentle movements or pressure. This increase in pain sensitivity reflects changes in the processing of sensory stimuli. Afferent nociceptor fibres are sensitized by the inflammatory process to the extent that the same stimulus produces much greater responses. Normally silent mechanoceptors are also sensitized and begin to respond to twisting and other mechanical stresses. These changes appear to be induced by cytokines produced in the inflamed joints. Sensitization also occurs in the spinal cord, with evidence that induced hyperexcitability of dorsal horn cells leads to amplification of nociceptive processing in the spine. The spinal changes appear to be induced both by altered afferent activity and by neuropeptides generated centrally. These changes in the peripheral and central nervous systems are called 'functional neuroplasticity'. Inflammation-induced changes sensitize afferent nociceptive fibres to mechanical, thermal, and chemical stimuli, converting nonpainful stimuli into painful ones.[12] Although NSAIDs help to control the pain, in the longer run this is insufficient, and disease-modifying drugs that halt or delay joint destruction are essential, not only to control short-term pain and stiffness but also to reduce joint destruction, which is the cause of so much pain and disability later in the course of the disease. The earlier use of these disease-modifying drugs, perhaps in combinations of several and preferably within the first 3–6 months of inflammatory polyarthritis, is thought to be necessary to reduce this damage for most individuals. There is concern, however, about how best to select those most at risk from those who will recover. Research into anticytokine and other newer agents (see Chapter 5) shows early promise, but the long-term effects are less clear.

Rheumatologists are accustomed to using means other than drugs to help their patients, but must now become adept at understanding not just physiotherapeutic techniques but also how to deal with the psychological and social factors which cause distress and disability. Coping is a psychological mechanism for managing stress. It involves changes of behaviour, thoughts or feelings.[13] In chronic illnesses, coping strategies attempt to mediate between the disease and its effects on the individual. As an individual adjusts to different stresses and to changes in a chronic disease, so their coping strategies may change. Through the course of RA, coping has to address an ever changing agenda, although pain and uncertainty are common features throughout its course. Not all coping mechanisms are adaptive or helpful. Furthermore, the ability of a person with RA to cope with their pain and disability is influenced strongly by mood, past experience and social circumstances. Pain and functional disability are rarely completely resolved and are important contributors to depression in the first few years of RA. An understanding of the individual's behavioural and emotional responses to the symptoms and the resultant disability in these early years may facilitate the design of interventions which will enhance the quality of life and avoid ineffective coping behaviours later on.[14] New therapeutic techniques, including care of the whole individual at an early stage of RA, demands early referral to a specialized and multiskilled team. Polyarthritis should be diagnosed and cared for by experts.

'WHIPLASH' INJURY

The term whiplash injury raises the spectre of serious medicolegal consequences. The majority of such injuries result from road traffic accidents in which the vehicle is hit from behind. Victims are affected differently according to how much warning they had of the impact and whether their body was fixed with a seat belt. The degree of pain and the length of time for which symptoms persist are apparently only partly related to the force of the impact and the immediate pain.[15] There is a strong impression that the way in which the problem is handled during its early stages by medical attendants and by the persons themselves is important in determining outcome. Adequate analgesia, support in a collar for a short time and sympathetic reassurance that the pain may last for a while but will eventually settle, all help. Lack of initial care, poor initial pain relief and anger are adverse factors in recovery. No-fault insurance may help. Often it is implied that the person is exaggerating the problem for profit. It is equally possible that the person becomes repeatedly reminded of their injury by interviews with lawyers and doctors during a long legal process and becomes frustrated and angry at the length of time that such litigation takes. Perhaps the process per se causes their chronic pain syndrome. 'Whiplash syndrome' is a difficult and frustrating process for the persons affected and for those who treat them.[16] More properly controlled research is needed and changes of attitudes by doctors, lawyers, and litigants are required if this difficult problem is to be resolved.

CHRONIC BACK PAIN

It is usual for most people to experience back pain at some time during their lives. As with other causes of pain, a simple somatic model of pain does not explain the nonlinear relationship between pain intensity and structural damage. Such variables as styles of thinking and ways of coping, levels of attention and distraction, beliefs about pain, and mood all have their effects. Any therapeutic approach that considers only a somatic approach is likely to be only partly effective. Indeed, it may be these psychological variables that are instrumental in converting acute episodes of pain into chronic pain syndromes. The physical approach to mechanical back pain is no longer to encourage bed rest until the pain has settled, but to encourage as near normal activity as possible, within the limits of tolerable pain. This produces a better short- to medium-term outcome than bed rest or specific exercises,[17] perhaps by decreasing the patient's focus on pain and disability.

Most people involved in the management of back pain, whatever their professional background, tend to think in terms of making a specific diagnosis and then adopting physical, pharmacological or surgical treatment regimes. Kerns and Jacob[18] have developed a model to explain why some people have a tendency to develop chronic pain. They suggest that congenital or acquired pre-existing susceptibilities or vulnerabilities such as abnormal thinking (cognitive), a tendency to anxiety (affective), a tendency always to go to bed when the pain is felt (behavioural) or factors in their social environment (social) may all predispose to the development of chronic pain. They suggest that abnormal thinking and increased pain behaviour associated with depression, fear and anxiety may combine to increase the likelihood of reduced physical activity due to the pain. When these factors are superimposed on other stresses created by the pain (anxiety, fear, physical impairment or perhaps physical changes in the CNS, for example), the experience of the back pain may persist or the degree of disability or distress is out of proportion to the structural changes that are detectable by the use of existing techniques.

If this model of chronic pain is correct, it implies that, even in early acute low back pain, recognition of the vulnerabilities of the individual and dealing with them are important therapeutic approaches that may actively prevent a transition to chronic back pain syndromes by targeting those individuals most at risk. Either the professionals managing back pain must broaden their approach or they must make more use of a multidisciplinary approach, which takes psychological and social management into account. Prevention is preferable to the challenge of managing a patient with a fully developed chronic pain syndrome, and the resultant disability and distress.

FIBROMYALGIA AND RELATED SYNDROMES

The definition of this complex syndrome, the nature and number of the trigger points, its relationship to such problems as irritable bowel syndrome, chronic fatigue syndrome, and tension headache, and the relevance of associated psychological factors such as anxiety and depression are the subject of considerable controversy. Some practitioners believe that it is a helpful diagnostic concept, while others find it hard to accept. These uncertainties are almost certainly due in part to the clear psychological dimension of the complaints which alienates some patients from their doctors. It is helpful to start from the viewpoint that fibromyalgia and the other dysfunctional disorders lie within a spectrum of diseases that includes major depressive disorders.[19] One of the difficulties with these disorders is that they cannot be diagnosed by tests; indeed, usually excessively extensive batteries of investigations prove to be normal. Fibromyalgia is best thought of as a core set of clinical features; palpable and reproducible tender points in a patient who complains of generalized muscular aching, stiffness, fatigue, and nonrestorative sleep comprise a recognizable pattern and lead to the diagnosis.[20] Some tests will be necessary to sort out the extensive differential diagnosis and to satisfy both the doctor and the patient that the diagnosis is correct. A variety of diverse treatment regimes have been tried. It may be possible to define distinct subgroups of patients with fibromyalgia by their psychological and behavioural characteristics and then tailor treatment more specifically.[21] Patients are helped by the recognition that their pain experience is subjective, by a positive approach to graded exercise, sometimes despite the pain, and by the cautious use of analgesics and tricyclic drugs, the latter in nonantidepressant doses. A nonjudgmental approach by the clinician is helpful, although often difficult to achieve.

There are some similarities between the so-called 'repetitive strain injuries' (RSI) and fibromyalgia. RSI usually arises in a work-related context and starts initially in the distal arm, but spreads in weeks or days to affect the whole limb. There are often trigger points similar to those seen in fibromyalgia; sleep patterns are disturbed, there are higher levels of anxiety and depression, and those affected have a strong belief in an underlying disease.[22] There appear to be few clear associations with specific work practices and more associations with psychosocial variables. Indeed, changes in the attitude of employers, especially immediate managers, doctors, physiotherapists, and employees are probably all keys to understanding the rise and fall of the epidemic of RSI in Australia. Important changes in workers' compensation schemes, where the first few treatments were not paid for and therefore had to be self-funded, were felt by many to have produced more change than any medical intervention.

REFLEX SYMPATHETIC DYSTROPHY

Reflex sympathetic dystrophy (RSD) is defined as: 'A descriptive term meaning a complex disorder or group of disorders that may develop as a consequence of trauma affecting the limbs, with or without obvious nerve lesions. RSD may also develop after visceral diseases, central nervous system lesions or, rarely, without an obvious antecedent event. It consists of pain and related sensory abnormalities, abnormal blood flow and sweating, abnormalities in the motor system and changes in structure of both superficial and deep tissues (trophic changes). It is not necessary that all components are present. It is agreed that reflex sympathetic dystrophy is used in a descriptive sense and does not imply specific underlying mechanisms'.[23] The length of this consensus statement demonstrates the problems that remain in defining and understanding the cause of this complex pain syndrome. The sympathetic, sensory, and motor changes are not confined to the zone of a single nerve and are generally distal. They do not necessarily occur in the region of injury, which may be unaffected. The problems of early recognition are real, but such recognition is essential to effective therapeutic treatment. The early symptoms of pain, generalized swelling, and a change of skin temperature may develop over a period of minutes or hours, usually quite soon after the initial insult. The fact that they are distal and distinct from the site of any initiating lesion are important diagnostic clues. This acute phase may develop, after a variable period of time, into a second or dystrophic stage, characterized by cold skin and trophic changes. Again after a further variable period of time, a third or atrophic phase, characterized by skin and muscle atrophy, bone changes and contractures may develop. Recovery is possible from the first two phases but not from the third. Specific tests such as a sympathetic block using local anaesthetic, the guanethidine test, and the phentolamine test may assist the diagnosis and be of prognostic value.[24] Treatment in the early stages may prevent progression and the development of a disorder that may cause years of pain, depression and disability. Early recognition and intervention in this rare but distressing disorder is infrequent, largely because general practitioners, orthopaedic surgeons, and others dealing with trauma are not sufficiently aware of it.

CONCLUSION

Some people with rheumatic disorders, despite treatment, live with intolerable pain. They have the right to expect treatment by a rheumatologist expert in all aspects of pain management. Often desperate and driven to rest excessively or to walk and move awkwardly by their pain, they are in a vicious circle of pain, fear, anxiety, and depression. They become unfit, weak, and increasingly isolated or dependent on others. They need to learn new ways to cope with their pain and keep on living a worthwhile and fulfilling life. Learning and then finding the courage to exercise despite the pain, to find other things to concentrate on besides the pain, and refocusing their thoughts away from the pain are all difficult, but not impossible, tasks. These can be achieved with help from a team which usually includes an interested doctor, a physiotherapist, and a psychologist. Whatever the cause of an individual's chronic pain syndrome, personal and environmental factors will have been essential elements in its development. These risk factors remain poorly researched. Indeed, the biological emphasis in the investigation of chronic pain syndromes may have done more harm than good by implying to the patient that all they have to do is to wait for the cure to arrive.[25] Rheumatologists can manage chronic pain better, not only by being expert in the use of a wide range of drugs and other pain-control techniques, but also by becoming involved in more longitudinal studies that focus specifically on psychosocial associations with the development of chronic pain and then by developing new approaches to its prevention. They owe it to their patients to become involved in multidisciplinary pain teams to which they can bring their experience of diagnosis and management to enhance the skills of anaesthetists, psychologists, physiotherapists, nurses, and social workers.

REFERENCES

1. Melzack R, Wall PD. Pain mechanisms: A new theory. *Science* 1965; **150**:971–8.
2. Woolf CJ. The dorsal horn. In: *Textbook of Pain* (Wall PD, Melzack R, eds.). Churchill Livingstone: Edinburgh, 1994:101–12.
3. Wall P D. Introduction. In: *Textbook of Pain* (Wall

PD, Melzack R, eds.). Churchill Livingstone: Edinburgh, 1994:1–7.

4. Melzack R. The McGill Pain Questionnaire: major properties and scoring methods. *Pain* 1975; **1**:277–99.
5. Craig KD, Prkachin KM. Non verbal measures of pain. In: *Pain Measurement and Assessment* (Melzack R, ed.). Raven Press: New York, 1983:173–82.
6. Keefe FO, Bradley L, Crisson JE. Behavioural assessment of low back pain: identification of pain behaviour subgroups. *Pain* 1990; **40**:153–60.
7. Wall PD. The placebo and the placebo response. In: *Textbook of Pain* (Wall PD, Melzack R, eds.). Churchill Livingstone: Edinburgh, 1994:1297–308.
8. Evans FJ. The placebo response in pain reduction. In: *Advances in Neurology* (Bonica JJ, ed.). Raven Press: New York, 1974:289–96.
9. Summers MN, Haley WE, Reveille JD, Alarcon GS. Radiographic assessment and psychologic variables as predictors of pain and functional impairment in osteoarthritis of the knee or hip. *Arthritis Rheum* 1988; **31**:204–9.
10. Dingle JT. The effect of NSAIDs on human articular cartilage glycosaminoglycan synthesis. *Eur J Rheumatol* 1996; **16**:47–52.
11. Gibson T, Clark B. Use of simple analgesics in rheumatoid arthritis. *Ann Rheum Dis* 1985; **44**:27–9.
12. Schaible HG. Why does an inflammation in the joint hurt? *Br J Rheumatol* 1996; **35**:405–6.
13. Lazarus RS. Stress, appraisal and coping, In: *Stress, appraisal and coping* (Lazarus RS, Folkman S eds). Springer Publications: New York, 1984:376–436.
14. Newman SP, Revenson T. Coping with rheumatoid arthritis. In: *Psychological Aspects of Rheumatic Diseases* (Newman SP, Shipley M eds.). Baillière Tindall: London, 1993; 7:259–80.
15. Radzanov BP, Sturzenegger M, Di-Stephano G. Long term outcome after whiplash injury. A 2-year follow-up considering features of injury mechanism and somatic, radiologic and psychosocial findings. *Medicine – Baltimore* 1995; **74**:281–97.
16. Pearce JMS. Whiplash injury – a reappraisal. *J Neurol Neurosurg Psychiatry* 1989; **52**:1329–31.
17. Malmivaara A, Hakkinen U, Aro T et al. The treatment of acute low back pain – bed rest, exercises or ordinary activity. *N Engl J Med* 1995; **332**:351–5.
18. Kerns RD, Jacob MC. Psychological aspects of back pain. In: *Psychological Aspects of Rheumatic Diseases* (Newman SP, Shipley M, eds.). Baillière Tindall: London, 1993; 7:337–56.
19. Hudson JI, Pope HG. The relationship between fibromyalgia and major depressive disorder. *Rheum Dis Clin North Am* 1996; **22**:285–304.
20. McCain GA. A cost effective approach to the diagnosis and treatment of fibromyalgia. *Rheum Dis Clin North Am* 1996; **22**:323–49.
21. Turk DC, Okifuji A, Sinclair D, Starz TW. Pain, disability and physical functioning – subgroups of patients with fibromyalgia. *J Rheumatol* 1996; **23**:1255–62.
22. Helme RD, LeVasseur SA, Gibson SJ. RSI revisited: evidence for psychological and physiological differences from an age, sex and occupation matched control group. *Aust NZ J Med* 1992; **22**:23–9.
23. Janig W, Blumberg H, Boas RA, Vampbell JA. The reflex sympathetic dystrophy syndrome. In: *Pain Research and Clinical Management 4* (Bonad MR, Charlton JE, Woolf CJ, eds.). Elsevier: Amsterdam, 1991:372–5.
24. Blumberg H, Janig W. Clinical manifestations of reflex sympathetic dystrophy and sympathetically maintained pain. In: *Textbook of Pain* (Wall PD, Melzack R, eds.). Churchill Livingstone: Edinburgh, 1994:685–98.
25. Carette S. Chronic pain syndromes. *Ann Rheum Dis* 1996; **55**:497–501.

7

Does the black population in Africa get SLE? If not, why not?

Ola Nived and Gunnar Sturfelt

The incidence and prevalence of rheumatic disorders in Africa are generally not very well studied. However, there is a prevailing opinion that systemic lupus erythematosus (SLE) is seldom seen, especially among the black populations of West Africa south of the Sahara. If this is true, it is in contrast to the consistently high incidence and prevalence of SLE observed in several black populations of the industrialized world.[1–3] This postulated discrepancy becomes even more intriguing when the ancestry is borne in mind of these populations, with their roots in West Africa some 200 years ago. At best such a difference in the epidemiological distribution of SLE could give the medical profession some clues to the aetiology or pathogenesis of the disorder. Formal studies performed with accepted epidemiological methodology are needed to settle the question definitely, but, as we still are lacking these studies, let us critically evaluate the available information to shed some light on the possible answers to the question: Does the black population in Africa get SLE? And, if not, why not?

SLE IN AFRICA

Olweny in 1961[4] published the first reported case of SLE in Africa – a man from Kenya in East Africa. During the following 10 years, case reports came from all parts of Africa. Subsequently the awareness of SLE has increased worldwide. This is indicated by an increasing number of publications, including some large series of African patients (Table 7.1). In Uganda only five SLE cases were reported initially,[5] but in 1980 a series of 21 cases was published.[6] In Zimbabwe in the 1960s no cases were seen during 5 years in Harare,[7] whereas 31 patients were reported from Bulawayo and Harare in 1986.[8] Over 300 cases have so far been reported from South Africa.[9–15] Apart from greater awareness, the improved availability and sensitivity of diagnostic laboratory facilities might be one cause for this observed increase in SLE. A further possibility advocated by some is a real increase in the incidence of SLE, a hypothesis that is hard to prove, since reliable epidemiological studies are lacking from previous years for comparison.

The publications concerning SLE in the black African population all have some findings in common. Firstly, more patients are found in urban than in rural areas. Secondly, most patients have severe organ manifestations. Thirdly, the mortality rate is high. These patterns of SLE are what might be expected in developing countries by comparison with reports from, for example, the populations of India and Brazil, and the Aborigines of Australia.[3,16–18] Unexpectedly, however, all series of African patients derive from northern, eastern or southern Africa. Up to 1996 only very few cases were reported from western Africa, including countries such as Nigeria, Côte d`Ivoire, and Gabon (Table 7.1, Figure 7.1). The reports of SLE in Africa are in parallel with the reports of rheumatoid arthritis (RA), another

Table 7.1 Reports of SLE in native African people by geographical region and country

Country	Observation period (years)	SLE cases in black population	Population	Reference	Year of publication
West Africa					
Nigeria	10 (1957–66)	2	Urban	Greenwood[28]	1968
Nigeria	1	1	Urban	Adebajo et al[46]	1992
Côte d'Ivoire	11	9	—	Monnier et al[47]	1985
Côte d'Ivoire	1	3	—	Lokrou et al[48]	1988
Gabon	—	1	—	Foruchet et al[49]	1969
Total reported		16			
East Africa					
Kenya	—	1	—	Olweny[4]	1961
Kenya	7 (1981–88)	67	Urban	Otieno et al[50]	1990
Ethiopia	—	15	—	Tsega et al[51]	1980
Zimbabwe	5	0	—	Gelfand[7]	1969
Zimbabwe	Retrospective	0	Rural	Lutalo[52]	1985
Zimbabwe	6	31	Urban	Taylor and Stein[8]	1986
Zimbabwe	—	20	—	Davis et al[53]	1989
Zimbabwe	0.5	18	Urban	Stein and Davis[54]	1990
Uganda	—	5	—	Shaper[5]	1961
Uganda	11	21	—	Kanyerezi et al[6]	1980
Total reported		188			
South Africa					
South Africa	11	8	Bantu	Jessop and Meyers[9]	1973
South Africa	7 (1969–75)	13	Zulu	Seedat and Pudifin[10]	1977
South Africa	15 (1970–84)	45	—	Morrison[11]	1988
South Africa	—	30	—	Dessein et al[12]	1988
South Africa	—	36	Urban	Sutej et al[13]	1989
South Africa	7 (1984–90)	85	Zulu	Mody et al[14]	1994
South Africa	—	49	—	Rudwaleit et al[15]	1995
Total reported		338			

diagnosis seldom made in the populations of West Africa.[19]

One possible reason for diagnosing SLE less often in one community than in another could be that the classification criteria, often used for diagnosis, do not apply in a special setting. Certainly this may be the case in parts of Africa. The specificity and sensitivity of the ACR criteria

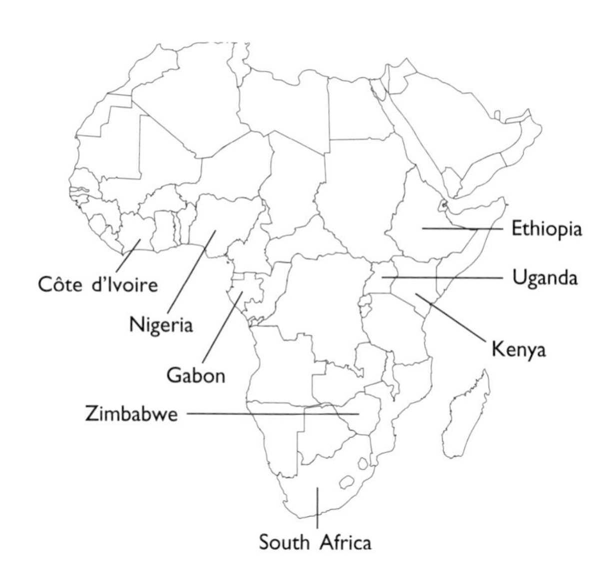

Figure 7.1 Map of Africa.

have been tested only in developed countries with mainly Caucasian populations, with low prevalence of infections, and a general absence of tropical diseases. Perhaps regional diagnostic criteria, as suggested by Adebajo,[20] are needed. Another possible reason could be that, despite an incidence approaching that seen in developed countries, the prevalence is kept low by a high mortality. High mortality could be caused by a deficient immune defence, leading both to SLE and to serious fatal infections, which may obscure the actual diagnosis of SLE.

However, if problems of criteria or high mortality were the main reasons for finding low frequencies of SLE in Africa during the 1960s, why has the number of reported cases subsequently increased in some parts of the continent but not in others? Have the countries of West Africa differed from the other countries of the continent with respect to development during the last 35 years? These questions are certainly

Table 7.2 Some demographic and social data from official national statistics of the countries in Table 7.1

Country	Population (millions)	Urban (%)	Infant mortality	Expected life span (years)	Physicians	Health care (% of national budget)
Nigeria	89 (1990)	35	98/1000	52	1/6400	3
Côte d'Ivoire	11.6 (1988)	43	110/1000	50	—	—
Gabon	1.1 (1988)	25	101/1000	51	—	—
Total	91.7					
Kenya	24.9 (1989)	—	72/1000	58	1/7200	5.2
Ethiopia	49.5 (1989)	—	Very high	47	—	—
Zimbabwe	10.7	—	—	59	—	—
Uganda	17.7	—	—	53	—	—
Total	102.8					
South Africa	37.7 (1991) (30 Africans)	43	53/1000	—	—	—
Total Africans	30					

difficult to answer. Urban areas are equally frequent in West and East Africa, and no consistent health care differences between these areas have been reported. Trained medical staff, well aware of SLE, are present in both East and West Africa (Table 7.2). Furthermore, as stated in a recent review by Symmonds,[21] the peoples of Africa have more genetic diversity than the rest of humankind put together, and the climate, environment, diet, and culture in that continent vary enormously.

Summing up the arguments above, we are still, in 1996, faced with a consistent lack of papers describing series of SLE patients in West Africa, which contrasts with the reported increased frequencies in other parts of Africa. Even with all the reservations stated above, we are still left with the notion that the prevalence of SLE in the black population of West Africa is extremely low. The prevalence is lower than in the rest of black Africans and in sharp contrast to the high incidence and prevalence consistently reported in Afro-Americans[1,2] and Afro-Europeans.[3] In fact, the incidence of SLE reported in black populations outside Africa is the highest reported in any populations. This highlights the hypothesis that different SLE distribution in the same race depends on geographical settlement.

All the available information for the moment thus supports the hypothesis of geographical differences, in addition to possible racial differences, but absolute proof of the hypothesis is lacking. Many other possible explanations exist. There are, for example, reports of genetic differences between black populations in Africa and the Afro-American population.[22] However, these studies are based on HLA alleles, not on haplotypes in families, and therefore conclusions about disease susceptibility cannot be drawn. Thus, we have a partial answer to the question posed by the title of this review. Some black populations in Africa seem to get SLE, some do not.

The evidence of differing incidences of SLE in Africa is fascinating, since it suggests the possibility of a hidden message for understanding basic disease mechanisms. This certainly warrants further analysis. Let us try to explore some possible factors that might give us clues about why SLE would be such a rare disorder in West Africa.

WHAT FACTORS DIFFER BETWEEN WEST AFRICA AND THE REST OF AFRICA?

Africa is a huge continent, the second largest in the world. It is divided by the equator, and the climate around this line is of course tropical, with subtropical areas to the north and south. West Africa south of the Sahara is part of the tropical region, but so also are parts of East Africa, from where series of SLE cases have been reported. Tropical climates per se do not seem to exclude the occurence of SLE. Comparisons with reports from tropical South America[23] and tropical Asia[24] do not support that conclusion either, but there are, of course, racial differences between these areas and Africa.

Topographically, Africa is divided into the northern lowlands and the southern highlands. The border between these areas with quite different living conditions runs from Ethiopia to northern Angola. This provides us with a difference, with East African SLE found in the highlands and West African SLE seemingly absent in the lowlands. The altitude is also of importance, for example, in modulating the climate, the vegetation, the wild-animal life, and the spectrum of infectious disorders.

Interestingly, epidemiologists have postulated that altitude is of importance for the incidence of RA in African black populations. This postulate is based on high frequencies of RA in some isolated high-altitude populations compared to low frequencies in some low-altitude populations.[25] This hypothesis has been somewhat contradicted by the reverse observation in Switzerland, but this latter report of course concerned Caucasians. With reference to SLE, a high prevalence is found in the tropical lowlands of Brazil,[23] and very large series of patients have been reported in the high-altitude capital of Mexico City.[26] However, these two reports emanate from overtly urban areas and do not include black populations.

The age-specific incidence of SLE differs, with the highest incidence occurring in young females of childbearing age in developing countries and a very low incidence found in prepubertal children. The fact that 45% of the black population of Africa is below the age of 15, and that in some areas the expected normal life span is less than 50 years, could account for some of the low frequencies noted (Table 7.2). Furthermore, severe forms of SLE with high mortality, resulting in low prevalences, might be expected in developing countries, on the basis of studies from other parts of the world.[18] However, the available data do not support the hypothesis of significant demographic differences with regard to length of life or infant mortality between West Africa and the rest of Africa. Examples of developing countries with high infant mortality and low life expectancy are found in both of these areas (Table 7.2).

Some notable demographic differences do exist between West Africa and the rest of Africa. In the north, east and south, Caucasians, e.g. Arabs and Indians, have to a much greater extent been resident (for centuries) than in the countries along the shores of the Gulf of Guinea. West Africa is still populated mostly by native Africans. In West Africa, the highest levels of polygamy are found, which is another difference from the rest of Africa.[27] Whether these facts have any bearing on the epidemiology of SLE is conjectural.

Without being able to exclude the possible influence of any of the above-mentioned background factors, we now change focus to an analysis of one of the most favoured hypotheses for an explanation of frequency differences of SLE in African black populations.

DO INFECTIONS IN WEST AFRICA INFLUENCE THE INCIDENCE OF SLE?

Greenwood postulated in 1968 that low frequencies of autoimmune disorders could be related to the presence of endemic parasitic infections, especially malaria.[28] This interesting suggestion can be divided into several possible different interactions, all of interest in a discussion of the epidemiology of SLE. Firstly, some infectious disorders might mimic SLE and thus could cause problems in differential diagnosis. Secondly, SLE patients have a reduced resistance to infection and this is a major cause of death in SLE.[18] Severe endemic infections might be rapidly fatal in patients with SLE, leading to a very low prevalence of SLE in the area affected. Thirdly, and most intriguingly, some infections might immunologically counteract the pathogenetic mechanisms that lead to SLE in the affected individual.

A plethora of infections cause major health problems for the populations of tropical Africa. It has been reported that some of these common endemic infections can pose differential diagnostic problems for SLE. Tuberculosis, in particular, can give rise to diagnostic confusion. The extrapulmonary manifestations of tuberculosis resemble many of the systemic manifestations of SLE.[29] Serositis in patients with SLE is, for example, often misdiagnosed as tuberculosis[10] and it is noteworthy that the original cutaneus manifestation named lupus vulgaris in the nineteenth century was actually due to cutaneous tuberculosis. The co-occurence of SLE and tuberculosis in the same patient is also common in Africa. This was the case in 10% of the Zimbabwean patients described by Taylor and Stein[8] and in 17% of the South African series of SLE published in 1988.[12] The autoantibody profile reported in patients with tuberculosis may also be a cause of confusion; 40% of the patients have antinuclear antibodies. These antibodies and others were also found in patients with many other tropical diseases. This topic has recently been reviewed in detail.[29] The situation of endemic tuberculosis in Africa thus might be a major explanation for misclassification of SLE.

Another infection causing differential diagnostic problems is HIV. HIV infection can cause lymphadenopathy, serositis, arthritis, skin rashes, neurological involvement, lymphopenia, thrombocytopenia, and increased antinuclear antibody titres.[30] However, the so-called 'AIDS belt', with the highest percentages of HIV cases, is located from southern Sudan, through Uganda, Tanzania, Zambia, Zimbabwe to Botswana in the south. Therefore, East and South Africa are affected to a greater extent than West Africa, causing the majority of differential diagnosis problems in these regions. The explosive spread of AIDS in these areas will obviously focus health care on problems other than SLE in the future, but it can also be expected to lead to many misclassified cases.

It is well known that patients with SLE are at increased risk for aquiring infections.[31,32] Infections are also one of the major causes of SLE fatalities worldwide.[18] Therefore, in developing countries with high frequencies of endemic infections, patients with SLE might be at risk of early fatal infections leading to a relatively low SLE prevalence. Of course, a genetically determined immune deficiency could be the common denominator for susceptibility to both SLE and infection. One such possible common denominator is genetically determined complement deficiency. This hypothesis needs to be studied further. It is not known whether the patients with SLE also have an increased risk of infection before the rheumatic disorder appears. If so, childhood infections might further reduce the incidence of SLE.

The third theory, of interaction between parasitic infections and autoimmunity, deserves special attention. When Greenwood, in his preliminary communication in 1968,[28] proposed the hypothesis, he focused on malaria. His findings were based on a study of polyarthritis in Nigeria and he was impressed by the extremely low frequency of autoimmune disorders among the admissions to the University Hospital in Ibadan. Out of 98 454 admissions during the period 1957 to 1966, only 104 patients with autoimmune disorders were found. Forty-two of these had RA, mostly seronegative, 21 had Still's disease, two had SLE and one had systemic sclerosis. None had primary myxoedema or Addison's disease, and no Africans had pernicious anaemia, all disorders well known in Afro-Americans. In this study an age-specific comparison was made with comparable hospital admissions in Britain: the Nigerian frequency of RA was one-sixth of that expected. Greenwood postulated that the rarity of autoimmune disease in western Nigeria, and possibly in other parts of tropical Africa, was similarly related to an altered immunological state produced by multiple parasitic infections since childhood, especially malaria. As evidence for this, it was pointed out that the gammaglobulin level in apparently healthy Africans was higher than that found in healthy Europeans or Afro-Americans. Part of the elevation of the gammaglobulins was due to antimalarial antibodies, and consequently antimalarial therapy lowered the gammaglobulins.[33] These initial observations and theories were later expanded.

POSSIBLE MECHANISMS OF INTERACTION BETWEEN INFECTIONS AND SLE

Cross reacting epitopes of antibodies produced in infections and autoantibodies in SLE patients have been described. Examples are antibodies against heat-shock protein 90, produced in malaria, candidiasis, and aspergillosis.[34] Antibodies produced by *Trypanosoma cruzi* in Chagas' disease cross react with human ribosomal P protein and, conversely, antiribosomal P protein antibodies from SLE patients cross react with the trypanosomes.[35] Antibodies against the basement membrane laminin are shared between SLE patients and filariasis-infected patients, but the specificities between the antibodies spontaneously produced in SLE and those found after infection seem to differ.[36] In studies on mice, antibodies to nuclear antigens, common to those found in SLE by immunoblot, could be found after schistosomiasis. This led to a hypothesis of bilharzia as a possible 'trigger' of SLE.[37] Interactions between tropical infections and SLE are theoretically possible, on the basis of immunological findings, but whether these results have any importance from the epidemiological perspective is still completely unknown.

With reference to the malaria theory of Greenwood, it has recently been proposed that a possible SLE-inhibiting mechanism could be the increased production of tumour necrosis factor-α (TNFα) seen in malaria.[38,39] Mice that were poor producers of TNFα and were prone to lupus nephritis were protected from nephritis by injections of TNFα[40]. In human SLE, some reports indicate that the patients have insufficient production of TNFα, perhaps genetically based on the TNFα genes within the MHC.[41] Other reports indicate normal TNFα concentrations in patients with SLE. Another possible interaction between the malaria plasmodium and SLE nephritis has been studied in the New Zealand black and white mice. Induction of natural, lupus nephritis-protective antibodies was achieved in the infected animals.[42] Furthermore, malaria-infected mice produce DNA-reactive antibodies that induce the nephritis of malaria, with immunochemical properties similar but not identical to those found in SLE.[43] Confirmation of epidemiological data comparing the spread of SLE and malaria is lacking. However, it is of note that no series of SLE patients has been reported from highly malaria-endemic areas in rural South East Asia, but the disease is common in malaria-free urban locations.

The HIV epidemic might also influence the frequency of SLE through immunological interactions. Epidemiological data from Africa, America and South East Asia do not support an inhibiting effect of HIV-1 infection on SLE. The two disorders occur simultaneously in the same populations in the same areas. Since HIV also induces TNFα production, this to some extent negates the malaria hypothesis given above. However, one interesting observation is worth mentioning. In the shadows of the HIV-1 epidemic in the 'AIDS belt' of Africa, there is a less well known HIV-2 epidemic. The HIV-2 epidemic is most prominent in West Africa, with the first case isolated in 1986.[44] This disease is more slowly fatal than HIV-1; the patients develop protective antiviral antibodies that lead to lower frequencies of HIV-1.[45] This epidemic is furthermore shared between humans and monkeys of the West African region, and might therefore have existed in the region for a long time. It is interesting to speculate that this infection might be linked to the low frequencies of autoimmune disorders in the area.

CONCLUSION

Reports of low frequencies of SLE reported from West Africa have still not been contradicted after more than 30 years of increasing knowledge. Therefore, it seems justified to conclude that SLE is a rare disorder, not in Africans but in Africans living in West Africa. Formal epidemiological studies are still lacking, to confirm the rather sporadic reports published to date. Genetic differences between black populations might be one explanation, environmental differences another. Urbanization and better treatment of infections could be related to the increasing incidence and prevalence of SLE. Whether there is a more direct mechanism linking certain infections and the pathogenesis of SLE cannot be concluded. However, studies of parasitic infections and retroviral endemics have initiated exciting hypotheses regarding possible connections between autoimmunity and microbes.

REFERENCES

1. Fessel WJ. Systemic lupus erythematosus in the community: incidence, prevalence, outcome and first symptoms: the high prevalence in black women. *Arch Intern Med* 1974; **134**:1027–35.
2. Nossent JC. Systemic lupus erythematosus on the Caribbean island of Curacao: an epidemiological investigation. *Ann Rheum Dis* 1992; **51**:1197–201.
3. Johnson AE, Gordon C, Palmer RG, Bacon PA. The prevalence and incidence of systemic lupus erythematosus in Birmingham, England: relationship to ethnicity and country of birth. *Arthritis Rheum* 1995; **38**:551–8.
4. Olweny CL. Systemic lupus erythematosus in a male Kenyan African. *Makevere Med J* 1961; **20**:L15–18.

5. Shaper AG. Systemic lupus erythematosus. *East Afr Med J* 1961; **38**:134–44.
6. Kanyerezi BR, Lutalo SK, Kigonya E. Systemic lupus erythematosus: clinical presentation among Ugandan Africans. *East Afr M J* 1980; **57**:274–8.
7. Gelfand M. Medical arthritis in African practice. *Central Afr J Med* 1969; **15**:131–5.
8. Taylor HG, Stein CM. Systemic lupus erythematosus in Zimbabwe. *Ann Rheum Dis* 1986; **45**:645–8.
9. Jessop S, Meyers OL. Systemic lupus erythematosus in Cape Town. *S Afr Med J* 1973; **47**:222–5.
10. Seedat YK, Pudifin D. Systemic lupus erythematosus in black and Indian patients in Natal. *S Afr Med J* 1977; **51**:335–7.
11. Morrison RA. Systemic lupus erythematosus: varying disease manifestations in patients from four ethnic groups in Johannesburg. MD Thesis, University of Johannesburg, 1988.
12. Dessein PHMC, Gledhill RF, Rossouw DS. Systemic lupus erythematosus in black South Africans. *S Afr Med J* 1988; **74**:387–9.
13. Sutej PG, Gear AJ, Morrison RCA et al. Photosensitivity and anti-Ro (SS-A) antibodies in black patients with systemic lupus erythematosus. *Br J Rheum* 1989; **28**:321–4.
14. Mody GM, Parag KB, Nathoo BC, Pudifin DJ, Duursma J, Seedat YK. High mortality with systemic lupus erythematosus in hospitalized African blacks. *Br J Rheumatol* 1994; **33**:1151–3.
15. Rudwaleit M, Tikly M, Gibson K, Pile K, Wordsworth P. HLA class II antigens associated with systemic lupus erythematosus in black South Africans. *Ann Rheum Dis* 1995; **54**:678–80.
16. Kumar A, Malaviya AN, Singh RR, Singh YN, Adya CM, Kakkar R. Survival in patients with systemic lupus erythematosus in India. *Rheumatol Int* 1992; **12**:107–9.
17. Anstey NM, Dunckley H, Bastian I, Currie BJ. Systemic lupus erythematosus in Australian Aborigines: high prevalence, morbidity and mortality. *Aust NZ J Med* 1993; **23**:645–53.
18. Nived O, Sturfelt G. Mortality in systemic lupus erythematosus. *Rheumatol Eur* 1996; **25**:17–19.
19. Adebajo AO, Reid DM. The pattern of rheumatoid arthritis in West Africa and comparison with a cohort of British patients. *Q J Med* 1991; **80**:633–40.
20. Adebajo AO. Epidemiology and community studies: Africa. *Baillerière's Clin Rheumatol* 1995; **9**:21–30.
21. Symmonds DPM. Lupus around the world, frequency of lupus in people of African origin. *Lupus* 1995; **4**:176–8.
22. Arnett FC, The genetic basis of lupus erythematosus. In: *Dubois' Lupus Erythematosus*, 4th edn (Wallace DJ, Hahn B, eds.). Lea & Febiger: Philadelphia, 1993:13–36.
23. Johnson AE, Cavalcanti FS, Gordon C et al. Cross sectional analysis of the differences between patients with systemic lupus erythematosus in England, Brazil and Sweden. *Lupus* 1994; **3**:501–6.
24. Frank AO. Apparent predisposition to systemic lupus erythematosus in Chinese patients in West Malaysia. *Ann Rheum Dis* 1980; **39**:266–9.
25. Moolenburgh JD, Valkenburg HA, Fourie PB. A population study on rheumatoid arthritis in Lesotho, Southern Africa. *Ann Rheum Dis* 1986; **45**:691–5.
26. Alarcon-Segovia D, Deleze M, Oria CV et al. Antiphospholipid antibodies and the antiphospholipid syndrome in systemic lupus erythematosus. A prospective analysis of 500 consecutive patients. *Medicine* 1989; **68**:353–65.
27. Caldwell JC, Caldwell P. The African AIDS epidemic. *Sci Am* 1996; **274**:40–6.
28. Greenwood BM. Autoimmune diseases and parasitic infections in Nigerians. *Lancet* 1968; **2**:380–2.
29. Adebajo AO, Isenberg DA. Immunological aspects. In: *Tropical Rheumatology*. Clinical Immunology Series (McGill PE, Adebajo AO, eds.). Baillière Tindall: London, 1995:215–29.
30. Mody GM. Rheumatoid arthritis and connective tissue disorders: sub-Saharan Africa. *Baillière's Clin Rheumatol* 1995; **9**:31–44.
31. Ginzler E, Diamond H, Kaplan D, Weiner M, Schlesinger M, Seleznick M. Computer analysis of factors influencing frequency of infection in systemic lupus erythematosus. *Arthritis Rheum* 1978; **21**:37–44.
32. Nived O, Sturfelt G, Wollheim FA. Systemic lupus erythematosus and infection. A controlled and prospective study including an epidemiological group. *Q J Med* 1985; **218**:271–87.
33. McGregor IA, Gilles HM. Studies on the significance of high serum gamma-globulin concentrations in Gambian Africans. II. Gammoglobulin concentrations of Gambian children in the fourth, fifth and sixth years of life. *Ann Trop Med Parasit* 1960; **54**:275–80.
34. al-Dughaym AM, Matthews RC, Burnie JP.

Epitope mapping human heat shock protein 90 with sera from infected patients. *Immunol Med Microbiol* 1994; **8**:43–8.

35. Skeiky YA, Benson DR, Guderian JA, Sleath PR, Parsons M, Reed SG. *Trypanosoma cruzi* acidic ribosomal P protein gene family. Novel P proteins encoding unusual cross-reactive epitopes. *J Immunol* 1994; **151**:5504–15.
36. Garcia Lerma J, Moneo I, Ortiz de Landazuri M, Sequi Navarro J. Comparison of the anti-laminin antibody response in patients with systemic lupus erythematosus (SLE) and parasitic diseases (filariasis). *Clin Immunol Immunopathol* 1995; **76**:19–31.
37. Rahima D, Tarrab-Hazdai R, Blank M, Arnon R, Shoenfeld Y. Anti-nuclear antibodies associated with schistosomiasis and anti-schistosomal antibodies associated with SLE. *Autoimmunity* 1994; **17**:127–41.
38. Adebajo AO. Does tumor necrosis factor protect against lupus in West Africans? *Arthritis Rheum* 1992; **35**:839.
39. Bate CAW, Taverne J, Playfair JHL. Soluble antigens are toxic and induce the production of tumor necrosis factor in vivo. *Immunology* 1989; **66**:600–5.
40. Jacob CO, McDewitt HO. Tumor necrosis factor-alfa in murine autoimmune 'lupus' nephritis. *Nature* 1988; **331**:356–8.
41. Jacob CO, Fronek ZI, Lewis GD, Koo M, Hansen JA, McDewitt HO. Heritable major histocompatibility complex class II-associated differences in production of tumour necrosis factor alfa: relevance to genetic predisposition to systemic lupus erythematosus. *Proc Natl Acad Sci USA* 1990; **87**:1233–7.
42. Hentati B, Sato MN, Payelle-Brogard B, Avrameas S, Ternynck T. Beneficial effect of polyclonal immunoglobulins from malaria-infected BALB/c mice on the lupus-like syndrome of (NZB × NZW) F1 mice. *Eur J Immunol* 1994; **24**:8–15.
43. Lloyd CM, Collins I, Belcher AJ, Manuelpillai N, Wozencraft AO, Staines NA. Characterization and pathological significance of monoclonal DNA-binding antibodies from mice with experimental malaria infection. *Infect Immun* 1994; **62**:1982–8.
44. Clavel F, Guétard D, Brun-Vezinet F et al. Isolation of a new human retrovirus from West African patients with AIDS. *Science* 1986; **223**:343–6.
45. Travers K, Mboup S, Marlink R et al. Natural protection against HIV-1 infection provided by HIV-2. *Science* 1995; **268**:1612–15.
46. Adebajo AO, Birell F, Hazleman BL. The pattern of rheumatic disorders seen amongst patients attending urban and rural clinics in West Africa. *Clin Rheum Dis* 1992; **11**:512–15.
47. Monnier A, Delmarre B, Peghini M et al. Le lupus erythemateux aigu dissemine en Côte-d'Ivoire (a propos de 9 observations). *Med Trop* 1985; **45**:47–54.
48. Lokrou A, Die-Kacou H, Toutou T et al. La maladie lupique: a Abidjan. A propos de 3 nouvelles observations. *Med Trop* 1988; **48**:65–7.
49. Foruchet M, Gateff C, Pineau J. Lupus erythemateux aigu dissemine chez l'Africain. A propos du premier cas observe au Gabon. *Med Trop* 1969; **29**:204–7.
50. Otieno LS, McLigeyo SO, Kayima JK, Sitati S. Management of lupus nephritis at the Kenyatta National Hospital. *East Afr Med J* 1990; **67**:387–95.
51. Tsega E, Choremi H, Bottazzo GF, Doniach D. Prevalence of autoimmune diseases and autoantibodies in Ethiopia. *Trop Geogr Med* 1980; **32**:231–6.
52. Lutalo SK. Chronic inflammatory rheumatic diseases in black Zimbabweans. *Ann Rheum Dis* 1985; **44**:121–5.
53. Davis P, Stein M, Ley H et al. Serological profiles in the connective tissue diseases in Zimbabwean patients. *Ann Rheum Dis* 1989; **48**:73–6.
54. Stein M, Davis P. Rheumatic disorders in Zimbabwe: a prospective analysis of patients attending a rheumatic disease clinic. *Ann Rheum Dis* 1990; **49**:400–2.

8

Does plasma exchange have any part to play in the management of SLE ?

Clare E McLure and David A Isenberg

Plasma exchange has been used for the treatment of systemic lupus erythematosus (SLE) for more than 20 years. After initial enthusiasm, its cost and doubts about its effectiveness have had an adverse effect upon its use. Recently, a large European study has led to re-evaluation of the utility of plasma exchange in SLE. In this chapter we look at how it is thought to work, review critically some of the important older papers and consider why plasma exchange is enjoying a revival in some quarters.

DEFINITION

Plasmapheresis, or plasma exchange, is the modern equivalent of blood-letting. It involves drawing blood from the patient, separating the plasma and returning the cellular components with replacement colloid to the patient.

TECHNIQUE

Plasma exchange became possible when cell separators were developed. More recently, membrane filtration devices have allowed removal of plasma from whole blood during extracorporeal perfusion.[1] Fresh frozen plasma, albumin and the purified protein fraction are used as colloid to replace the patient's plasma. The benefits and side-effects of plasmapheresis are influenced by the type of replacement fluid, the volumes of fluid exchanged, and the frequency of the procedure: 4-litre plasma exchange removes 95%, and 2-litre removes 75% of an intravascular marker.[2] Volume replacement with complement-containing fluid may lessen the tendency for immune complexes to be deposited in tissues and may enhance the clearance of immune complexes, as there are receptors for C3b on mononuclear phagocytes.[3] However, infusion of complement-free fluid may also be beneficial, as complement is an important mediator of damage caused by immune complexes and autoantibodies.

SIDE-EFFECTS

The incidence of side-effects from plasmapheresis varies between 10%[4] and 40%.[5] Severe reactions are rare (1%).[4] The incidence of fatal complications varies between 0.05%[4] and 0.2%.[5] There is a higher incidence of side-effects in severely ill patients, in those with multisystem disease, and in centres which only rarely perform plasmapheresis.[5,6] In centres with considerable experience, plasmapheresis is generally well tolerated in adults. Common complications include transient hypotension, problems related to the need for vascular access, and reactions to citrate anticoagulation. The last is a result of a reduction in the level of ionized calcium as a result of chelation, and usually causes parasthesaie. Problems of vascular access and general acceptability of the procedure are, on the whole, much greater in children and adolescents. Rare problems include syncope, cramps, abdominal and back pain, local infection, transfusion-related infection, peripheral nerve trauma, air embolus, haemolysis, bleeding due to depletion of coagulation components or platelets, or sometimes the converse – the formation of clots. Haemodynamic complications include acute cardiac insufficiency, acute lung injury, myocardial ischaemia, and arrythmia. Hypersensitivity reactions may occur.[7] Side-effects vary, depending on the replacement fluid used. For example, hypersensitivity reactions are most likely when fresh frozen plasma is administered, and, in oliguric patients, fluids containing sodium citrate are likely to result in severe alkalosis.

THEORETICAL CONSIDERATIONS

Many of the clinical features in SLE have been considered to be attributable to the deposition of immune complexes. Subsequent activation of complement and other mediators of inflammation results in tissue damage.[8] Autoantibodies also directly cause damage, as has been confirmed recently by a study in which hybridomas producing IgG anti-double-stranded DNA antibodies were grown in SCID mice and were shown to induce proteinuria.[9] Autoantibodies may also play a part in the loss of suppression by T cells, which results in B-cell hyperactivity. By decreasing the concentration of immune complexes, autoantibodies, complement system components, and mediators of inflammation, plasma exchange is thought to interrupt and temporarily suppress the chain of pathological events leading to tissue damage in SLE.

Levels of immune complexes are decreased by plasmapheresis in some patients to a greater extent than would be expected from the volume of plasma removed. This may be due to improvement of the functioning of the mononuclear phagocytic system, simply by a reduction in the immune complex load being processed by the overburdened liver and spleen.[10] However, other factors may be involved, for example alteration of the physical properties of the complexes (size, charge, etc) and changing membrane receptor function.[11] Work with heat-damaged red blood cells and autologous IgG-coated erythrocytes has demonstrated that splenic hypofunction correlates with lupus disease activity and levels of circulating immune complexes. The hyposplenism was reversed completely by plasma exchange within about 48 hours, as disease activity and levels of immune complexes decreased.[12,13]

Immune function is affected in other ways by plasma exchange. Short-term observations include improvement of bacterial killing by monocytes,[14,15] decrease in anti-T suppressor cell antibodies, anti-precursor cell antibodies,[16–18] and antibody-blocking E-rosette receptors.[17] Increase in T suppressor cells and decrease in the CD4/CD8 ratio has been noted following plasma exchange.[19] Idiotype–anti-idiotype relationships are also affected.[20]

Klippel has suggested that the biological consequences of plasma exchange are likely to be far-reaching.[11] Changes in hormones, cell membrane function, cellular secretions, and regulatory processes probably all result. There are shifts between intra- and extravascular compartments with the establishment of new equilibria and compensatory changes in synthetic and catabolic rates of depleted factors.

Klippel also commented that the observed biological changes might be due to the plasmapheresis process itself and not because of the components removed.[11] Intermittent anticoagulation with heparin or citrate dextrose solution will produce numerous changes. Contact with the surface of tubing is likely to result in activation of certain biological systems; for example, complement and platelet activation.[21] Cell membrane characteristics may be affected. Properties of blood vessels are altered by factors such as depletion of vasoactive peptides and decrease in plasma viscosity.

Use of fresh frozen plasma as a replacement solution provides plasma constituents that may be useful; for example, clotting factors, beneficial for conditions such as thrombotic thrombocytopenic purpura or the haemolytic uraemic syndrome (which can occasionally occur as complications of SLE), or complement in people with congenital deficiency of a complement component.

Theoretically, there may be detrimental as well as beneficial effects of plasma exchange. Mediators helping to counteract tissue damage may be removed.[18] Following plasma exchange, 'antibody rebound' tends to occur, due to a loss of negative feedback.[22,23] This is partially clone-specific and may be due to the removal of feedback inhibition by anti-idiotype antibodies and immune complexes. B cells proliferate and antibody levels increase to more than their pre-exchange level. Campion has pointed out that removal of plasma or lymphocytes will not eliminate tissue antigen, and has little effect on high-affinity autoantibodies, immune complexes, and activated T cells in tissues.[18] Local production of antibody or mediators of inflammation may be unaffected or even increased.

The experimental and clinical findings of a regulatory effect of circulating antibodies on the synthesis of antibodies of the same specificity[24–30] led to the concept of synchronization or synchronized deletion.[31] This involved utilization of plasmapheresis to stimulate rebound proliferation of clone-specific lymphocytes. Proliferating B cells are maximally sensitive to immunosuppressives, so large doses could then be administered to kill the pathogenic clones.[26,31–33] Experimental work supports this mechanism.[22] Administration of cytotoxic drugs following selective removal of antibody in dogs has been shown to produce prolonged and profound specific reduction in antibody synthesis.[25]

CLINICAL STUDIES

Jones et al[34] first used plasma exchange in SLE in 1976. It appeared to be promising. There followed a series of reports of improvement following plasma exchange for virtually every manifestation of SLE and this included life-threatening, steroid-resistant problems.[31,32,35–39]

However, virtually all studies shared a major problem with 'antibody rebound' – temporary relief was followed by a rapid increase in autoantibodies and flare of disease activity if no or only low-dose immunosuppression accompanied the plasma exchange.[31,40] Efficacy was well established for certain disease subsets, such as thrombotic thombocytopenic purpura,[41] cryoglobulinaemia, and the hyperviscosity syndrome.[42] However, the early studies were not controlled and, in general, the indications for plasma exchange remained unclear in the early 1980s.

Controlled studies subsequently showed disappointing results, when plasma exchange was compared with immunosuppression alone. Long-term oral immunosuppression was combined with plasma exchange in these trials. A summary of the features is presented in Table 8.1. Wei et al[43] conducted a small but well controlled, double-blind trial comparing 20 patients with mild active lupus randomized to receive either plasma exchange over 2 weeks or sham apheresis. Oral steroids were used, but not cytotoxic drugs. The patients only had six plasma exchanges over a 2-week period and had a short follow-up period of just 6 weeks. There was a significant reduction in serum immunoglobulins and circulating immune complexes, but no difference in clinical response. As the authors pointed out, this negative result does not rule out a beneficial effect for plasmapheresis, because their numbers were so small.

The French Co-operative Group[44] compared the short-term effect of plasma exchange with steroids in the treatment of severe lupus flares, and found no difference in outcome. They treated patients with severe active SLE, but excluded those with rapidly progressive glomerulonephritis. Patients were followed for 29 months, but 46% of their patients were withdrawn, mainly because of deteriorating health. Hence, their conclusion that the two groups had the same outcome was based on analysis of only 12 patients.

Lewis et al[45] looked at 86 patients with severe lupus nephritis randomized to be given short-term high-dose oral cyclophosphamide and steroid plus or minus 10 plasma exchanges over 1 month. They had a long follow-up period,

Table 8.1 Features of controlled studies on plasma exchange

Study	No. of patients	Disease features	Treatment before plasma exchange	Exchanges	Controls	Treatment after plasma exchange	Follow-up	Results
Wei et al (1983)[43]	20	Mildly active SLE	15 on steroids (mean dose 15 mg/day). No cytotoxics	6 × 41 exchanges over 2 weeks. Normal saline replacement	Sham apheresis	15 on steroids. 5 NSAIDs/hydroxy-chloroquine	6 weeks	No difference between 2 groups. 16 no change/improved. 2 worse. 2 withdrawn because of disease exacerbation (1 plasmapheresed, 1 not)
Clark et al (1984)[48]	39	Diffuse proliferative glomerulo-nephritis	Steroids ± azathioprine. 7 patients not on cytotoxics	41 exchanges. Active disease: 5× in 2 weeks then 1× every 3–4 weeks. Inactive disease: 1× every 3–4 weeks. 5% albumin or plasma replacement	No exchanges	Adjustment of previous regime. Increased steroids ± azathioprine if disease active, and vice versa	3 years	No difference between groups
French Co-operative Group (1985)[44]	25	Severe active SLE	?	60 ml/kg exchanges. 5× in 1st week. 6× during next 2 weeks. 2× per week for 23 sessions. 4% albumin replacement	No exchanges	1.5 mg/kg per day for 60 days, then decreased to reach 1 mg/kg per day at day 90	29 months	No difference between groups. 46% withdrawn, mainly because of deteriorating condition

Wallace et al (1988)[47]	27	Nephrotic syndrome – classes III/IV/V lupus nephrits (82% proliferative 18% membranous)	Failed to respond to treatment with steroids + cytotoxics	40 ml/kg exchanges. 12× over 4 weeks. Albumin replacement	No exchanges	Continued on previous regime. 85% on alkylating agent	2 years	7 'good responders' (creatinine normalized and no longer had nephrotic syndrome) – all plasmapheresed. 13 no change. 7 'poor responders' (serum creatinine >3 mg/dl, death or end-stage renal failure) – 5 were plasmapheresed
Lewis et al (1992)[45]	86	Severe lupus nephritis – classes III/IV/V	?	<55 kg (31). >55 kg (41). 10× over 4 weeks. Albumin replacement	No exchanges	All received 60 mg prednisolone + 2 mg/kg oral cyclophosphamide/ day for 4 weeks. If improvement clinically, tapering of cyclophosphamide over 4 weeks + prednisolone over 22 weeks. Prednisolone continued at 20 mg alternate days. If SLE worse/persistent activity/reappearance, more intensive drug regime, then return to the withdrawal protocol	Mean of 136 weeks. Extended to over 5 years	No significant difference between groups

SLE, systemic lupus erythematosus; NSAIDs, nonsteroidal anti-inflammatory drugs with a mean of 136 weeks, (extended to 5 years). Despite a substantial decrease in the serum concentration of antibodies against double-stranded DNA and cryoprecipitable immune complexes, and immunosuppression sufficient to prevent rebound of autoantibody production following plasma exchange, there was no difference in the outcome between the two groups. However, most of the important endpoints occurred long after the 4-week plasmapheresis phase. Therefore, it may be difficult to attribute the results in the plasmapheresis group to the exchange procedure itself.[46]

Wallace et al[47] found modest benefits only. They looked at 27 patients with lupus nephritis resistant to 3 months' immunosuppression. All patients continued their 'pretreatment' steroid and immunosuppressive regime and 17 patients had 12 plasma exchanges over a 4-week period. Their plasma was exchanged on one of two different machines (a cell separator and a selective membrane device), and there was a lack of standardization of the concomitant immunosuppressive therapy. Seven of the patients who had plasma exchange had a good response, whereas none of the ten control patients did. However, there was no change in the clinical condition of 13 patients, and seven responded poorly, five of whom were plasmapheresed.

Clark et al[48] found subgroup-related benefit only, in a randomized, controlled trial of 39 patients with SLE and diffuse proliferative glomerulonephritis. They were randomized to receive long-term plasma exchange and 'conventional therapy' vs conventional therapy alone. These investigators were studying a different subgroup of patients from those in Wallace's smaller study, as their patients had not 'failed' conventional therapy. Their immunosuppressive therapy was not standardized. Seven patients received just steroids, 32 received azathioprine as well. Immunosuppressive doses were adjusted during the study, according to disease activity. They had a relatively long follow-up period of 3 years. When the results were analysed with exclusion of the nine Jamaican patients, they were able to show improvement for patients treated by plasma exchange compared with controls. Their exclusion was felt to be justified, because of the geographic and racial differences in the severity of SLE and because those patients received volume replacement with plasma rather than albumin. However, there was no significant difference in outcome when all the patients were included in the analysis.

In general, those patients most seriously ill seemed to benefit most from plasma exchange.[35,49] From these trials it was concluded that in mild SLE there was no indication for plasma exchange. Even in most cases of diffuse proliferative glomerulonephritis, plasma exchange offered no advantage over conventional therapy that used steroids and cyclophosphamide. However, there appeared to be a place for it in subsets of patients; for example, those with renal disease who were resistant to steroid and cytotoxics, and in hyperviscosity, thrombotic thrombocytoperic purpura (TTP), cryoglobulinaemia, and the acute life-threatening complications of SLE.[50] It was generally agreed that concomitant immunosuppression should be used.[7]

The technique of synchronized deletion followed from the experience of using plasma exchange without concomitant immunosuppression – rebound increase in the level of autoantibodies and immune complexes followed the initial deletion, and an increase in disease activity accompanied this.[20,35,40] As indicated above, the idea centred on the enhancement of the cytotoxic drug effect by stimulation of autoreactive lymphocytes with plasma exchange. Schroeder et al[51] used this technique and reported rapid improvement of disease activity in two patients with severe SLE who had not responded to conventional therapy. They were given large volume plasma exchange followed by intravenous cyclophosphamide, then low-dose oral cyclophosphamide for a further 6 months. The patients' disease remained inactive after 14 months of follow-up. Dau et al[52] used the technique on a patient with severe SLE. Following six monthly cycles of plasma exchange with synchronized cyclophosphamide, the SLE went into remission, accompanied by not only a decrease in the concentrations of circulating B and T lymphocytes, but also a decrease in the ratio of CD4 to CD8 cells. CD8+ DR+ CDw29+ suppressor/ cytotoxic T cells increased, and the percentage of the CD4+ CD45R+ T helper cells decreased. The activated memory phenotypes of the cytotoxic suppressor population might have played a role in the control of the autoreactive B and T cells, and hence of disease activity.

The most convincing use of synchronized deletion has come from the study by Euler et al.[53] Immunosuppression was withdrawn from 14 patients with severe SLE. Large-volume, short-interval pulses of plasmapheresis were given, 4% human albumin used as the replacement solution. This was followed by high dose (12 mg/kg) cyclophosphamide during the assumed period of clonal vulnerability. The patients then received 6 months of oral cyclophosphamide and prednisolone therapy. There was a rapid improvement in all patients. At 6 months 12 out of 14 patients had achieved clinical remission and were able to stop immunosuppressives. Clinical remission had been maintained in eight of the 14 patients without immunosuppressives for 7 years, and in some for up to 9 years.[46] The T4/T8 ratio was markedly decreased by the plasmapheresis and cyclophosphamide, and continued for 2–3 years. However, as the T4/T8 ratio gradually rose back to normal, there was no accompanying increase in disease activity. Euler and Guillevin concluded that synchronization may have induced normalization of the immune system.[54]

Euler's group felt that there were certain key points in their protocol. Immunosuppressives were decreased before and during plasmapheresis, in order to ensure the maximum cytotoxic effect of the cyclophosphamide on fully activated lymphocytes. Antibody was then extensively removed by short-interval, large-volume plasma exchange. Albumin was used as a replacement solution to avoid passive administration of antibody, which might blunt the stimulus to lymphocyte proliferation.[29,55] A dose of pulsed cyclophosphamide, 20–40% higher than previously used in rheumatic disease, was then administered during the period when the lymphocyte clones were felt most likely to be at their most 'vulnerable'. Immunosuppression was maintained after the pulsed cyclophosphamide with oral cyclophosphamide and steroid to prevent the reactivation of pathogenic clones.

Other groups have subsequently used the same protocol in a nonrandomized trial. An interim analysis of 24 patients revealed that six of the patients had died. Four of the deaths were due to fulminant lupus or late complications of SLE, and two were due to infection. The Lupus Plasmapheresis Study Group felt that patients who were unsuitable for this protocol may have been recruited, so discontinued this open part of their study (JO Schroeder, personal communciation).

Concern has been expressed about the mortality rate due to infection following the synchronization technique. However, Euler's group and the Steglitz Clinic in Berlin have treated 25 patients with the original protocol, without any deaths from infection.[56] The Lupus Plasmapheresis Study Group are conducting an international multicentre randomized trial[54] with the use of a modified form of the original synchronization protocol; 151 patients have been randomized. The study is in its final evaluation phase and results are expected to be published in late 1996/1997. A panel of experts studied the clincial results and data relevant to therapeutic safety in April 1994, and recommended continuation of the study (JO Schroeder, personal communication).

Synchronization of plasmapheresis with subsequent intravenous immunoglobulin has also been shown to result in short-term improvement.[57,58] This may be useful for patients with severe SLE and sepsis, but is unlikely to result in more than temporary benefit.[46]

IMMUNOADSORPTION

Selective removal of specific plasma proteins is now possible with membrane filtration or immunoadsorbent columns. For example, cryoproteins,[59] anti-single-stranded DNA,[60] anti-double-stranded DNA,[61] lupus anticoagulant, and anti-cardiolipin antibodies[62] have all been removed selectively. More selective removal of fluid requiring smaller volumes of replacement fluid would permit larger volumes of blood to be processed and provide a significant cost benefit. However, membranes activate complement and may present additional risks of haemolysis.[50]

There are case reports of the successful use of specific immunoadsorbent columns.[63,64] It has been shown that highly selective adsorption of a particular antibody does not induce rebound of the same antibody and may be followed by long-term suppression of antibody synthesis. This may be because counter-regulatory anti-idiotypes are not removed.[65] However, there are a number of problems associated with the use of columns that adsorb specific antibodies. It is not known precisely which antibodies to target, because our understanding of the pathogenesis of SLE is not sufficiently advanced. A number of different autoantibodies are probably involved in the disease process. Therefore, removal of a single autoantibody is unlikely to be helpful. In addition, the heterogeneous nature of individual types of antibody (for example, against double-stranded DNA) in terms of their antigen specificity, affinity, and avidity[66] means that the use of specific immunoadsorption appears to be limited at present.

Double-column systems that remove all types of immunoglobulin look more promising.[46] In these systems one column elutes while the other adsorbs. The process is lengthy and expensive, but enables a large volume of plasma to be processed with a higher rate of antibody depletion than in plasmapheresis. At present, however, the place of these systems in the management of the disease remains unclear.

CONCLUSIONS

Although a decade ago plasma exchange seemed best reserved as a last ditch treatment for a 'desperate disease', the recent work with the technique of 'synchronized deletion' suggests that a revival may be at hand. There is no indication for the use of plasma exchange in patients with mild or moderately active disease. However, it may yet become part of the management of some patients with severe SLE, although further large trials are needed to establish its place. The key beneficial effect of plasma exchange is not the removal of harmful substances per se, but the resultant stimulation of the proliferation of pathogenic lymphocyte clones. Proliferating lymphocytes are maximally vulnerable to cytotoxic drugs. Hence, plasmapheresis increases the effectiveness of immunosuppressive therapy. If the early work on synchronization can be reproduced, plasmapheresis followed by cyclophosphamide could result in prolonged disease remission. It is expensive and not without risk – patients will be very susceptible to infection after plasma exchange and large doses of cytotoxics, but in certain restricted circumstances plasma exchange may have a place in the treatment of severe SLE.

REFERENCES

1. Shumak KH, Rock GA. Therapeutic plasma exchange. *N Engl J Med* 1984; **310**:762–71.
2. Takahashi M, Czop J, Ferreira A, Nussenzweig V. Mechanism of solubilization of immune aggregates by complement: implications for immunopathology. *Transplant Rev* 1976; **32**:121–39.
3. Lockwood CM, Rees AJ, Pearson TA, Evans DJ, Peters DK, Wilson CB., Immunosuppression and plasma exchange in the treatment of Goodpasture's syndrome. *Lancet* 1976; **i**:711–5.
4. Mokrzycki MH, Kaplan AA. Therapeutic plasma exchange: complications and management. *Am J Kidney Dis* 1994; **23**:817–27.
5. Belloni M, Alghisi A, Scremin L. Complications of plasma exchange. *Int J Artif Organs* 1993; **16** (Suppl 5):180–2.
6. Bussel A, Pourrat J, Elkharrat D, Gajdos P. The

French registry for plasma eschange: a four year experience. *Int J Artif Organs* 1991; **14**:393–7.
7. Council on Scientific Affairs. Current status of therapeutic plasmapheresis and related techniques. *J Am Med Assoc* 1985; **253**:819–25.
8. Brentjens J, Ossi E, Albini B. Disseminated immune deposits in lupus erythematosus. *Arthritis Rheum* 1977; **20**:962–8.
9. Ehrenstein MR, Katz DR, Griffiths M et al. Human IgG antiDNA antibodies deposit in kidneys and induce proteinuria in SCID mice. *Kidney Int* 1995; **48**:705–11.
10. Hamburger MI, Gerardi EN, Fields TR, Bennett RS. Reticulo-endothelial system Fc function and plasmapheresis in systemic lupus erythematosus. *Artif Organs* 1981; **5**:264–8.
11. Klippel JH. Apheresis, Biotechnology and the rheumatic diseases. *Arthritis Rheum* 1984; **27**:1081–5.
12. Frank MM, Hamburger MI, Lawley TJ, Kimberley RIP, Plotz PH. Defective Fc receptor function in lupus erthematosus. *N Engl J Med* 1979; **300**:518–23.
13. Lockwood CM, Worlledge S, Nicholas S, Cottoc C, Peters DK. Reversal of impaired splenic function by plasma exchange, *N Engl J Med* 1979; **300**:524–30.
14. Nihei N, Fukuma N, Ohashi Y et al. Effects of plasmapheresis on immunological status in systemic lupus erythematosus. In: *Proceedings of the First International Congress of the World Apheresis Association: Therapeutic Plasmapheresis.* ISAO Press: Cleveland, 1987:623–6.
15. Steven MM, Tanner AR, Holdstock GE et al. The effect of plasma exchange on the in vitro monocyte function of patients witn immune complex diseases. *Clin Exp Immunol* 1981; **45**:240–5.
16. Abdou NI, Lindsley HB, Pollock A, Stechschulte DJ. Plasmapheresis in active systemic lupus erytmematosus: effects on clinical serum and cellular abnormalities. Case report. *Clin Immunol Immunopathol* 1981; **19**:44–54.
17. Morimoto D, Reinherz EL, Abe T, Homma M, Schlossman SF. Characteristics of anti-T cell antibodies in systemic lupus erythematosus: evidence for selective reactivity with normal suppressor cells defined by monoclonal antibodies. *Clin Immunol Immunopathol* 1980; **16**:474–84.
18. Campion EW. Desperate diseases and plasmapheresis. *N Engl J Med* 1992; **326**:1425–7.
19. Vangelista A, Frasca GM, Nanni-Costa A, Bonomini V. Effects of plasmapheresis on E-rosette receptors in systemic lupus erythematosus patients. *J Clin Apheresis* 1986; **3**:100–2.
20. Zouali M, Eyquem A. Idiotype anti-idiotype interactions in SLE. *Ann Immunol* 1983; **134C**:377–91.
21. Zielinski CC, Wolf A, Eibl MM. Plasapheresis for rheumatoid arthrits. *N Engl J Med* 1983; **309**:986–7.
22. Bystryn JC, Scherkein I, Uhr JW. A model for regulation of antibody synthesis by serum antibody. In: *Progress in Immunology* (Amos B, ed.). Academic Press: New York, 1971.
23. Euler HH, Schroeder JO. Antibody depletion and cytotoxic drug therapy in severe systemic lupus erythematosis. *Transfusion Sci* 1992; **13**:167–84.
24. Brystryn JC, Graf MW, Uhr JW. Regulation of antibody formation by serum antibody: II. Removal of specific antibody by means of exchange transfusion. *J Exp Med* 1970; **132**:1279–87.
25. Terman DS, Gracia-Rinaldi R, Dannemann B et al. Specific suppression of antibody rebound after extracorporeal immunoadsorption: I. Comparism of single versus combination chemotherapeutic agents. *Clin Exp Immunol* 1978; **34**:32–41.
26. Euler HH, Krey U, Schroeder O, Loffler H. Membrane plasmapheresis technique in rats: confirmation of antibody rebound. *J Immunol Methods* 1985; **84**:313–19.
27. Sturgull BC, Worzniak MJ. Stimulation of proliferation of 19s antibody forming cells in the spleens of immunized guinea pigs after exchange transfusion. *Nature* 1970; **228**:1304–5.
28. Uhr JW, Baumann JB. Antibody formation: I. Suppression of antibody formation by passively administered antibody. *J Exp Med* 1961; **113**:935–57.
29. Chang H, Schneck S, Brody NI, Deutsch A, Sisund GW. Studies on the mechanism of the suppression of active antibody synthesis by passively administered antibody. *J Immunol* 1969; **102**:37–41.
30. Pierce CW. Immune response in vitro: II. Suppression of the immune response in vitro by specific antibody. *J Exp Med* 1969; **130**:365–79.
31. Jones JV. Plasmapheresis in SLE. *Clin Rheum Dis* 1982; **8**:243–60.
32. Jones JV, Robinson MF, Parciany RK, Layfer LF, McLeod B. Therapeutic plasmapheresis in systemic lupus erythematosus: effect on immune complexes and antibodies to DNA. *Arthritis Rheum* 1981; **24**:1113–20.

33. Parry HF, Moran CJ, Snaith ML et al. Plasma exchange in SLE. *Ann Rheum Dis* 1981; **40**:224–8.
34. Jones JV, Brucknall RC, Cumming RH, Asplin CM. Plasmapheresis in the management of SLE. *Lancet* 1976; **i**:709–11.
35. Jones JV, Cumming RH, Bacon PA et al. Evidence for a therapeutic effect of plasmapheresis in patients with systemic lupus erythematosus. *Q J Med* 1979; **48**:555–76.
36. Jones JV, Clough JD, Klinenberg JR, Davis P. The role of plasmapheresis in the rheumatic diseases. *J Lab Clin Med* 1981; **97**:589–98.
37. McKenzie PE, Taylor AE, Woodroffen AJ, Seymour AE, Chan YL, Clarkson AR. Plasmapheresis in glomerulonephritis. *Clin Nephrol* 1979; **12**:97–108.
38. Ibister JP, Ralston M, Wright R. Fulimant lupus pneumonitis with acute renal failure and red blood cell aplasia. Successful management with plasmapheresis and immunosuppression. *Arch Intern Med* 1981; **141**:1081–5.
39. Wysenbeek AJ, Smith JW, Krakauer RS. Plasmapheresis II: Review of clinical experience. *Plasma Ther Transfusion Technol* 1981; **2**:61–71.
40. Schlansky R, De Horatius PJ, Pincus T, Tung KSK. Plasmapheresis in systemic lupus erythematosus: a cautionary note. *Arthritis Rheum* 1981; **24**:49–53.
41. Rock GA, Shumak KH, Buskard NA et al. Comparison of plasma exchange with plasma infusion in the treatment of thrombotic thrombocytopenic purpura. *N Engl J Med* 1991; **325**:393–7.
42. Wallace DJ, Klinenberg JR. Apheresis. *Dis Mon* 1984; **30**:1–45.
43. Wei N, Klippel JH, Huiston DP et al. A randomized trial of plasma exchange in mild systemic lupus erythematosus. *Lancet* 1983; **i**:17–21.
44. French Co-operative Group. A randomized trial of plasma exchange in severe acute systemic lupus erythematosus: methodology and interim analysis. *Plasma Ther Transfusion Technol* 1985; **6**:535–9.
45. Lewis EJ, Hunsicker LG, Lan SP, Rohde RD, Lachin JM, for the Lupus Nephritis Collaborative Study Group. A controlled trial of plasmapheresis in severe lupus nephritis. *N Engl J Med* 1992; **326**:1373–9.
46. Euler HH, Zeuner RA, Schroeder JO. Plasma exchange in systemic lupus erythematosus. *Transfusion Sci* 1996; **17**:245–65.
47. Wallace DJ, Golfinger D, Savage G et al. Predictive value of clinical, laboratory, pathologic and treatment variables in steroid/ immunosuppressive resistant lupus nephritis. *J Clin Apheresis* 1988; **4**:30–4.
48. Clark WF, Balfe JW, Cattran DC et al. Long-term plasma exchange in patients with SLE and diffuse proliferative glomerulonephritis. *Plasma Ther Tranfusion Technol*; 1984; **5**:353–60.
49. Jones JV. Plasmapheresis in JLE. *Clin Rheum* 1982; **8**:243–60.
50. Wallace DJ, Non-pharmacologic therapeutic modalities. In: *Dubois' Lupus Erythematosus*, 4th edn. (Wallace DJ, Hahn BH, eds.). Lea & Febiger: Philadelphia, 1993: 958–9.
51. Schroeder JO, Euler HH, Loeffler H. Synchronization of plasmapheresis and pulse cyclophosphamide in severe systemic lupus erythematosus. *Ann Intern Med* 1987; **107**:344–6.
52. Dau PC, Callahan J, Parker R, Golbus J. Immunologic effects of plasmapheresis with pulse cyclophosphamide in systemic lupus erythematosus. *J Rheumatol* 1991; **18**:270–6.
53. Euler HH, Schroeder JO, Harten P, Zeuner RA, Guitschmidt HJ. Treatment-free remission in severe systemic lupus erythematosus following synchronization of plasmapheresis with subsequent pulse cyclophosphamide. *Arthritis Rheum* 1994; **37**:1784–94.
54. Euler HH, Guillevin L. Plasmapheresis and subsequent pulse cyclophosphamide in severe systemic lupus erythematosus. An interim report of the Lupus Plasmapheresis Study Group. *Ann Med Intern* 1994; **145**:296–302.
55. Rossi F, Jayne DRW, Lockwood CM, Kazatchkine MD. Anti-idiotypes against anti-neutropohil cytoplasmic antigen autoantibodies in normal human polyspecific IgG for therapeutic use and in remission sera of patients with systemic vasculitis. *Clin Exp Immunol* 1991; **83**:298–303.
56. Euler HH, Moeller J, Schroeder JO. Synchronization with subsequent pulse cyclophosphamide in SLE [abstract]. *Lupus* 1995; **4** (Suppl 2):112.
57. Francioni C, Galeazzi M, Fioravanti A, Gelli R, Megale F, Marcolong R. Longterm IV Ig treatment in systemic lupus erythematosus. *Clin Exp Rheumatol* 1994; **12**:163–8.
58. Pirner K, Rubbert A, Burmester GR, Kalden JR, Manger B. Intravenous administration of immunoglobulins in systemic lupus erythematosus: review of the literature and initial clinical

experiences. *Infusionsther Transfusionsmed* 1993; **20** (Suppl 1):131–5.
59. Koo AP, Segal AM, Smith JW, Smith DS, Krakauer RS. Continuous flow cryofiltration in the treatment of systemic vasculitis [abstract]. *Arthritis Rheum* 1983; **26** (Suppl):S67.
60. Terman DS, Buffalo G, Mattioli C et al. Extracorporeal immunoadsorption: initial experience in human SLE. *Lancet* 1979; **ii**(8147):824–7.
61. El Habib R, Laville M, Traeger J. Specific adsorption of circulating antibodies by extracorporeal plasma perfusions over antigen coated collagen flat-membranes: application to systemic lupus erythematosus. *J Clin Lab Immunol* 1984; **15**:111–17.
62. Tsuda H, Taniguchi O, Mokuna C. Utilization of dextran sulphate column plasmapheresis to remove anti-cardiolipin antibodies. *Jap J Artif Organs* 1989; **18**:7–10.
63. Kinoshita M, Aotsika S, Funahashi T, Tani N, Yokahari R. Selective removal of anti-double stranded DNA antibodies by immunoadsorption with dextran sulphate in a patient with systemic lupus erythematosus. *Ann Rheum Dis* 1989; **48**:856–60.
64. Kobayashi S, Tamura N, Tsuda H, Mokuna C, Hashimoto H, Hirose S. Immunoadsorbent plasmapheresis for a patient with anti-phospholipid syndrome during pregnancy. *Ann Rheum Dis* 1992; **561**:399–401.
65. Zeuner RA, Beress R, Schroeder JO, Euler HH. Effect of antigen-specific immunoadsorption on antibody kinetics in a rat model. *Biomater Artif Cells Artif Organs* 1993; **21**:199–211.
66. Smeenk RJ, van Rooijen A, Swak TJ. Dissociation studies of DNA/anti-DNA complexes in relation to anti-DNA avidity. *J Immunol Methods* 1988; **109**:27–35.

9

Is mixed connective tissue disease a myth?

Frank HJ van den Hoogen and Leo BA van de Putte

INTRODUCTION

The term connective tissue disease (CTD) was introduced by Klemperer, Pollack, and Baehr in 1942.[1] A number of disease entities were integrated into this term, with heterogeneous involvement of various organs and with fibrinoid degeneration of the connective tissue as the common morphological feature. The most prominent CTDs at that time were systemic lupus erythematosus disseminatus (SLE) and systemic sclerosis (scleroderma); other diseases such as dermato/polymyositis (DM/PM) and Sjögren's syndrome also became part of the CTD family. It soon appeared that these diseases shared more than just morphological features. There is a clear preference for the female sex and age of onset of disease during the childbearing years, and it turned out that in most of the patients with a CTD autoantibodies could be detected. Connective tissue is present in every organ, and in CTDs every organ can be involved in the disease process, either simultaneously or sequentially. In addition, CTDs are characterized by overlap of symptoms. In order to differentiate the various CTDs from other diseases and from each other, much effort was put into the classification of the CTDs. These classifications depended on the recognition of certain clinical characteristics and/or laboratory tests. Classification criteria were established for SLE in 1971[2] and revised in 1982,[3] for systemic sclerosis[4] and recently for Sjögren's syndrome.[5] Criteria for the diagnosis of DM/PM, proposed by Bohan et al,[6] are applied widely. These classification and diagnostic criteria have gained worldwide acceptance and have helped in the standardization of clinical studies. They have also contributed to earlier recognition of disease, better understanding of its natural history and occurrence of complications, and to the determination of the most optimal treatment. However, these classifications are blurred by the presence of overlapping and transitory forms.

Table 9.1 Clinical characteristics of 25 patients with mixed connective tissue disease (after Sharp et al[7])

Characteristic	Frequency (%)
Arthralgias	96
Arthritis	68
Raynaud's phenomenon	88
Abnormal oesophageal motility	77
Myositis	72
Lymphadenopathy	68
Fever	32
Hepatomegaly	28
Serositis	24
Splenomegaly	21
Renal disease	0
Anaemia	48
Leukopenia	52
Hypergammaglobulinaemia	80

Table 9.2 Preliminary diagnostic criteria for mixed connective tissue disease (MCTD)

	Requirements for diagnosis of MCTD
Sharp[10] A. Major criteria 1. Myositis, severe 2. Pulmonary involvement (a) CO diffusing capacity <70% normal (b) Pulmonary hypertension (c) Proliferative vascular lesion or lung biopsy 3. Raynaud's phenomenon or oesophageal hypomotility 4. Swollen hands observed or sclerodactyly 5. Highest observed anti-U1RNP ≥ 1 : 10000 Minor criteria 1. Alopecia 2. Leucopenia 3. Anaemia 4. Pleuritis 5. Pericarditis 6. Arthritis 7. Trigeminal neuropathy 8. Malar rash 9. Thrombocytopenia 10. Myositis, mild 11. Swollen hands	Definite (a) 4 majors anti-U1RNP ≥ 1 : 4000 Probable (a) 3 majors and anti-U1RNP ≥ 1 : 1000 (b) 2 majors from 1,2 and 3 and 2 minors with anti-U1RNP ≥ 1 : 1000 Possible (a) 3 majors (b) 2 majors and anti-U1RNP ≥ 100 (c) 1 major and 3 minors and anti-U1RNP ≥ 1 : 100
Kasukawa et al[11] A. Common symptoms 1. Raynaud's phenomenon 2. Swollen fingers or hands B. Anti-U1RNP antibody C. Mixed findings (a) SLE-like findings 1. Polyarthritis 2. Lymphadenopathy 3. Facial erythema 4. Pericarditis or pleuritis 5. Leucopenia or thrombocytopenia	1. Positive in either of 1 of 2 common symptoms 2. Anti-U1RNP antibody 3. Positive in 1 or more findings in C2 or 3 disease categories or (a), (b), and (c)

(b) SSc-like findings
1. Sclerodactyly
2. Pulmonary fibrosis, restrictive change of lung or reduced diffusion capacity
3. Hypomotility or dilatation of oesophagus

(c) PM-like findings
1. Muscle weakness
2. Increased serum levels of myogenic enzymes (CPK)
3. Myogenic pattern in EMG

Alarcón-Segovia and Villarreal[12]

1. Serological: positive anti-U1RNP at a haemagglutination titre of 1 : 11600 or higher	1. Serological
2. Clinical: Oedema of the hands Synovitis Myositis Raynaud's phenomenon Acrosclerosis	2. At least three clinical data 3. The association of oedema of the hands, Raynaud's phenomenon and acrosclerosis requires at least one of the other two criteria

CO, carbon monoxide; ENA, extractable nuclear antigens; RNP, ribonucleoprotein; CPK, creatine phosphokinase; PM, polymyositis; SLE, systemic lupus erythematosus; EMG, electromyogram; SSc, systemic sclerosis.

In each of these diseases recognition of groups of clinical symptoms antedated the recognition of linked antibodies. In contrast, Sharp and colleagues initially identified anti-ribonucleoprotein (RNP) RNP-positive patients and then tried to demonstrate that these individuals had similar clinical features.

Thus, in 1972 Sharp et al[7] described a syndrome, which was called mixed connective tissue disease (MCTD). It was clinically denoted by features of two or more defined autoimmune CTDs, namely SLE, systemic sclerosis and DM/PM, and the presence of a high titre of circulating antibodies to an RNAse-sensitive extractable nuclear antigen. This antigen proved to be a RNP that plays an important role in premessenger RNA splicing[8] and is composed of a small nuclear (sn) RNA designated U1, and three or more distinct U1-RNA binding proteins.[9] Antibodies directed against the (U1)snRNP (anti-(U1)snRNP antibodies) are considered to be the hallmark of MCTD. Apart from the anti-(U1)snRNP antibodies, other characteristics of MCTD were stated to be infrequent renal, pulmonary and cerebral involvement, good response to low doses of corticosteroids and a favourable prognosis. However, since the first description, the concept of MCTD as a truly distinct disease entity has been questioned in many reports. Therefore, the issue to be considered is: what, if anything, discriminates MCTD from the other well-classified connective tissue diseases?

IS MCTD CLINICALLY DISTINCT FROM OTHER CTDS?

Clinical and laboratory features of the first 25 patients with MCTD, as reported by Sharp and co-workers,[7] are listed in Table 9.1. The most common clinical characteristics were severe arthralgias, diffusely swollen hands, Raynaud's phenomenon, oesophageal dysmotility, myositis and lymphadenopathy. Frank arthritis was present in 68%; although most of these patients had nondeforming arthritis, three patients had arthritic features resembling rheumatoid arthritis (RA). Haematological abnormalities consisted of anaemia, leukopenia and hypergammaglobulinaemia. All these clinical and laboratory features are common manifestations of rheumatic disorders and cannot be considered to be unique pathognomic characteristics of MCTD. Moreover, combinations of these manifestations also occurred in patients without anti-(U1)snRNP antibodies. When it became clear that the original definition of MCTD could not be maintained, several attempts were made at a better definition of MCTD. Three different sets of criteria were proposed[10–12] (Table 9.2), all requiring a combination of nonspecific clinical symptoms with or without anti-(U1)snRNP antibodies for the diagnosis of MCTD. When these three different sets of criteria were tested in patients with well-defined CTDs, including MCTD, it was found that the sets of criteria fared similarly in capturing nearly all 'so-called' MCTD patients, but that they fared less well in ruling out patients with other CTDs, especially systemic sclerosis.[13] This lack of specificity prevents the application of these criteria in clinical practice.

Initially it was stated that clinically apparent pulmonary, renal, and neurological involvement in patients with MCTD was rare, that vasculitis did not occur, and that symptoms responded dramatically to low doses of glucocorticoids. However, since then a number of reports have stressed the relatively frequent occurrence of serious complications, including pulmonary, renal, neuropsychiatric, and cardiovascular diseases, and vasculitis.[14–18] These complications were often so severe that administration of high doses of glucocorticoids and even cytostatic drugs was considered to be necessary. Even then, a fatal outcome could not always be prevented. Reviewing five series of MCTD patients, Black and Isenberg[19] noted that 13% of the patients had died after a mean disease duration of 12 years[20–24] (Table 9.3). The impression of MCTD as a benign disease was thus refuted by these observations.

Several follow-up studies have been performed in patients with an initial diagnosis of MCTD. Nimelstein et al[22] re-evaluated the original 25 patients of Sharp and colleagues. After 8 years of follow-up, 17 patients were re-examined. Systemic sclerosis was diagnosed in 10 patients (including one with coexisting RA and one with SLE), RA and SLE were diagnosed in one each, and five patients were asymptomatic. Lundberg et al[25] observed a development towards SLE in only one out of 17

Table 9.3 Prognosis in five series of patients with mixed connective tissue disease, with sequential evaluations (after Black and Isenberg[19])

Number studied	Deaths	Mean duration of disease (years)	Reference
100	4	6	Sharp et al[20]
15	4	6.8	Singsen et al[21]
22	8	12	Nimelstein et al[22]
23	5	?	Grant et al[23]
34	4	11	Sullivan et al[24]
194	25 (13%)		

patients with MCTD after a mean observation period of 65 months; none developed symptoms compatible with systemic sclerosis, DM/PM or RA. In contrast, De Clerck et al[26] found that 70% of 18 patients diagnosed as suffering from MCTD evolved to SLE or systemic sclerosis after a mean duration of follow-up of 4.6 years. Similar results were obtained by Van den Hoogen et al:[27] after a follow-up period of 2.6 years after the first clinical presentation, 55% of the patients initially diagnosed as suffering from MCTD could be classified as having SLE, systemic sclerosis, RA or a combination of these diseases. The anomalous results of these studies might be explained by different classifications of MCTD at study entry. It appears, however, that a substantial number of patients with anti-(U1)snRNP antibodies in whom, at presentation, no diagnosis (according to the well-established criteria for SLE, systemic sclerosis, DM/PM or RA) can be made, may subsequently develop signs and symptoms that will allow such diagnoses to be established.

CAN MCTD BE DISCRIMINATED EPIDEMIOLOGICALLY FROM OTHER CTDS?

The female preponderance of MCTD is just as marked as in other CTDs: approximately 80% of the patients are females.[28] MCTD mostly starts during the childbearing years,[28] but it can occur at any age, even in childhood.[21] No exact data on the prevalence of MCTD are known, but MCTD is considered to occur as frequently as systemic sclerosis, more commonly than polymyositis, and less frequently than SLE.[22] No particular racial or ethnic distribution has been noted, and no racial differences in expression of MCTD have been reported. Therefore, it seems that from an epidemiological point of view MCTD behaves like any other CTD.

IS MCTD SEROLOGICALLY DIFFERENT FROM OTHER CTDS?

Anti-(U1)snRNP antibodies are directed against an antigen composed of a small nuclear (sn) RNA designated U1, which is associated with a number of common proteins as well as with three distinct U1-snRNA binding proteins, namely U1-70K, U1-A, and U1-C.[9] Sera containing anti-(U1)snRNP antibodies have been found to react primarily with the 70-kDa and A protein, and also at a lower frequency with the C protein,[29] as well as with the U1snRNA.[30]

From the start, the presence of anti-(U1)snRNP antibodies was fundamental to the concept of MCTD as a separate disease entity. However, it soon transpired that these autoantibodies were not uniquely restricted to MCTD, but could also occur in every well-defined CTD. They have been shown in patients with SLE,[31–34] systemic sclerosis,[31–33] DM/PM,[31–33] and RA.[32,33] Occasionally, anti-(U1)snRNP antibodies have been reported in other autoimmune diseases.[35]

Anti-(U1)snRNP antibody titres can change with time,[25] and in some studies it was demonstrated that in some patients anti-(U1)snRNP antibodies can even disappear.[26,36] Titres of anti-U1snRNP antibodies do not appear to have a predictive value for disease activity; studies examining a possible relationship between titres and disease activity are hampered by difficulties in both quantitation of anti-U1snRNP antibodies and proper assessment of disease activity. Although in one study the fall or disappearance of anti-U1snRNP antibodies seemed to occur in association with prolonged remission,[37] other studies failed to demonstrate a correlation of anti-U1snRNP antibody titre and disease activity as determined by predefined criteria.[38,39] In one prospective study major disease exacerbations seemed to be associated with peaks in anti-U1snRNA antibody level.[40]

Antibodies to the 70-kDa, A and C proteins of the U1snRNP complex all contribute to the anti-U1 RNP response (Table 9.4). Antibodies to the 70-kDa component of the U1snRNP particle are detectable in most patients with MCTD, but have also been described in patients with SLE.[37,41,42] In patients with MCTD, preselected because of the presence of anti-U1snRNP antibodies, antibodies to the 70-kDa protein occur in 75–95%; anti-70-kDa antibodies can be detected in 12% of patients with SLE and

Table 9.4 Occurrence of antibodies directed to individual snU1RNP components in rheumatic diseases (after Craft and Hardin[46])

	MCTD	SLE	RA	SSc	DM/PM
anti-70-kDa protein	75–95%	12%	rare	rare	rare
anti-A protein	75–95%	23%	rare	rare	rare
anti-C protein	75–95%	23%	rare	rare	rare

MCTD, mixed connective tissue disease; SLE, systemic lupus erythematosus; RA, rheumatoid arthritis; SSc, systemic sclerosis; DM/PM, dermato/polymyositis.

occasionally in patients with RA, DM/PM or systemic sclerosis.[42] Interestingly, several studies have shown that the absence of antibodies specific for the 70-kDa band in patients with antibodies to U1snRNP particles is strongly associated with SLE.[37,41–45]

Antibodies to the A protein occur with the same frequency as anti-70-kDa antibodies in patients with MCTD, and were found in 23% of patients with SLE.[46]

Antibodies to the C protein are detected at approximately the same frequency as anti-70-kDa and anti-A antibodies in patients with MCTD and SLE; anti-A or anti-C antibodies are rare in RA, DM/PM or systemic sclerosis.[46]

Antibodies to the snU1RNA component of the U1snRNP particle have been found in 38% of patients with anti-U1snRNP antibodies.[30] The anti-U1snRNA antibodies were always accompanied by anti-U1snRNP antibodies;[30] peaks in anti-U1snRNA antibody titers seemed to be associated with major disease exacerbations.[40]

In many patients, antibodies other than anti-(U1)snRNP antibodies appear to be present at first clinical presentation.[27] These autoantibodies include rheumatoid factor and anti-dsDNA antibodies, and occasionally anti-centromere, anti-Sm, anti-Ro and anti-La antibodies.[27] In some patients, although these antibodies were not present at clinical presentation, they appeared during long-term follow-up.[27] It seems clear that none of the antibodies directed against any component of the ribonucleoprotein complex is specific for any of the CTDs, including MCTD.

GENETICS: IS MCTD GENETICALLY DIFFERENT FROM OTHER CTDS?

Patients with MCTD are reported to have a higher incidence of DR4 compared with normal controls,[47] but this increase appears to be restricted to the subgroup of patients with polyarthritis;[48] in this subgroup, there was no increased frequency of rheumatoid factor. It therefore seems likely that the observed association is related more to polyarthritis in general than to MCTD. The presence of anti-U1snRNP antibodies reacting with the 70-kDa protein was found to be associated with HLA-DR4/HLA-DRw53 or HLA-DR2.[49,50]

Several studies have examined immunoglobulin allotypes in patients with anti-U1snRNP antibodies. A strong association was found between the Km(1) phenotype and a susceptibility to SLE.[51] In one study the association with the Gm (1,3;5,21) allotype was reported,[52] but this was not confirmed in another study.[48]

An association of the MHC antigens was found with the evolution of MCTD: progression into systemic sclerosis was associated with HLA-DR5, and nondifferentiation was associated with

HLA-DR2 or DR4;[36] erosive and/or deforming arthritis was associated with HLA-DR1 or DR4. At present, no clearcut HLA association with MCTD is known.

CONCLUDING REMARKS

The dispute concerning the concept of MCTD as a distinct disease entity continues. The lack of sufficient data to confirm or undermine the concept has made this dispute one between ardently opposed believers and nonbelievers, and no decision can be made about whether MCTD should be considered to be a reality or a myth. One could argue that no disease entity has any right to exist, when 25 years after its first description, its concept is still heavily disputed. On the other hand, it cannot be ignored that a diagnosis of MCTD is still made by many physicians in patients with anti-(U1)snRNP antibodies and symptoms suggestive of a CTD, who cannot be diagnosed according to the classification criteria of any of the CTDs. Especially when only mild symptoms are present, it is satisfactory to both patients and physicians that a diagnosis such as MCTD, albeit much contested, can be made. Physicians are therefore tempted to tag patients with the diagnosis of MCTD, instead of waiting for specific features of any of the well-classified CTDs, which develop in most of the patients in due time.

The proposal to use the term undifferentiated connective tissue disease (UCTD) in undifferentiated autoimmune rheumatic disease, for those patients who do not fulfil the well-established classification criteria for a single CTD, until such time as they do so, might unite believers and nonbelievers, and change a myth into reality. This proposal, first put forward by LeRoy et al[53] and supported by others,[19,54] assumes that most of the patients with anti-(U1)snRNP antibodies finally develop a CTD. This concept of UCTD is more flexible than the concept of MCTD; patients with UCTD can be considered to be in a transient phase towards the development of a CTD. The broad acceptance of the concept UCTD, however, has to be accompanied by the funeral of the myth of MCTD. Until this is accomplished, the myth of MCTD lingers on.

REFERENCES

1. Klemperer P, Pollack AD, Baehr G. Diffuse collagen disease. Acute disseminated lupus erythematosus and diffuse scleroderma. *J Am Med Assoc* 1942; **119**:331–2.
2. Cohen AS, Reynolds WE, Franklin EC et al. Preliminary criteria for the classification of systemic lupus erythematosus. *Bull Rheum Dis* 1971; **21**:643–8.
3. Tan EM, Cohen AS, Fries JF et al. The 1982 revised criteria for the classification of systemic lupus erythematosus. *Arthritis Rheum* 1982; **25**:1271–7.
4. Masi AT, Rodnan GP, Medsger AT Jr et al. Preliminary criteria for the classification of systemic sclerosis (scleroderma). *Arthritis Rheum* 1980; **23**:581–90.
5. Vitalli C, Bombardieri S, Moutsopoulos HM et al. Preliminary criteria for the classification of Sjögren's syndrome. *Arthritis Rheum* 1993; **36**:340–7.
6. Bohan A, Peter JB, Bowman RL. Polymyositis and dermatomyositis. *N Engl J Med* 1975; **292**:344–7.
7. Sharp GC, Irvin WS, Tan EM, Gould RG, Holman HR. Mixed connective tissue disease – an apparently distinct rheumatic disease syndrome associated with a specific antibody to an extractable nuclear antigen (ENA). *Am J Med* 1972; **52**:148–59.
8. Steitz JA, Black DL, Gerke V et al. Functions of the abundant U-snRNPs. In: *Structure and Function of Major and Minor Small Nuclear Ribonucleoprotein Particles* (Birnstiel ML, ed.). Springer Verlag: Heidelberg, 1988:115–54.
9. Lührmann R. snRNP proteins. In: *Structure and Function of Major and Minor Small Nuclear Ribonucleoprotein Particles* (Birnstiel ML, ed.). Springer Verlag: Heidelberg, 1988:71–99.
10. Sharp GC. Diagnostic criteria for classification of MCTD. In: *Mixed Connective Tissue Diseases and*

Anti-nuclear Antibodies (Kasukawa R, Sharp GC, eds.). Elsevier: Amsterdam, 1987:23–32.

11. Kasukawa R, Tojo T, Miyawaki S et al. Preliminary diagnostic criteria for classification of mixed connective tissue disease. In: *Mixed Connective Tissue Diseases and Anti-nuclear Antibodies* (Kasukawa R, Sharp GC, eds.). Elsevier: Amsterdam, 1987:41–7.
12. Alarcón-Segovia D, Villarreal M. Classification and diagnostic criteria for mixed connective tissue diseases. In: *Mixed Connective Tissue Diseases and Anti-nuclear Antibodies* (Kasukawa R, Sharp GC, eds.). Elsevier: Amsterdam, 1987:33–40.
13. Alarcón-Segovia D, Cardiel MH. Comparison between 3 diagnostic criteria for mixed connective tissue disease. Study of 593 patients. *J Rheumatol* 1989; **16**:328–34.
14. Derderian SS, Tellis CJ, Abbrecht PH, Welton RC, Rajagopal KR. Pulmonary involvement in mixed connective tissue disease. *Chest* 1985; **88**:45–8.
15. Koboyashi S, Magase M, Kimura M, Ohyama K, Ikeza M, Honda N. Renal involvement in mixed connective tissue disease. *Am J Nephrol* 1985; **5**:282–7.
16. Bennett RM, Bong DM, Spargo BH. Neuropsychiatric problems in mixed connective tissue disease. *Am J Med* 1978; **65**:955–62.
17. Oetgen WJ, Mutter ML, Lawless OJ, Davia JE. Cardiac abnormalities in mixed connective tissue disease. *Chest* 1983; **83**:185–188.
18. Benett RM, O'Connell DJ. Mixed connective tissue diseases. A clinicopathologic study of 20 cases. *Semin Arthritis Rheum* 1980; **10**:25–51.
19. Black C, Isenberg DA. Mixed connective tissue disease – Goodbye to all that. *Br J Rheumatol* 1992; **31**:695–700.
20. Sharp GC, Irvin WS, May CM et al. Association of antibodies to ribonucleoprotein and Sm antigens with mixed connective-tissue disease, systemic lupus erythematosus and other rheumatic diseases. *N Engl J Med* 1976; **295**:1149–54.
21. Singsen BH, Bernstein BH, Kornreich HK, Koster King K, Hanson V, Tan EM. Mixed connective tissue disease in childhood. A clinical and serologic survey. *J Pediatr* 1977; **90**:893–900.
22. Nimelstein SH, Brody S, McShane D, Holman HR. Mixed connective tissue disease: a subsequent evaluation of the original 25 patients. *Medicine* 1980; **59**:239–48.
23. Grant KD, Adams LE, Hess EV. Mixed connective tissue disease – a subset with sequential clinical and laboratory features. *J Rheumatol* 1981; **8**:587–98.
24. Sullivan WD, Hurst DJ, Harmon CE et al. A prospective evaluation emphasizing pulmonary involvement in patients with mixed connective tissue disease. *Medicine* 1984; **63**:92–107.
25. Lundberg I, Nyman U, Pettersson I, Hedfors E. Clinical manifestations and anti-(U1)snRNP antibodies: a prospective study of 29 anti-RNP antibody positive patients. *Br J Rheumatol* 1992; **31**:811–17.
26. De Clerck LS, Meijers KAE, Cats A. Is MCTD a distinct entity? Comparison of clinical and laboratory findings in MCTD, SLE, PSS, and RA patients. *Clin Rheumatol* 1989; **8**:29–36.
27. Van den Hoogen FHJ, Spronk PE, Boerbooms AMT, Bootsma H, de Rooij DJRAM, Kallenberg CGM, Van de Putte LBA. Long-term follow-up of 46 patients with anti-(U1)snRNP antibodies. *Br J Rheumatol* 1994; **33**:1117–20.
28. Sharp GC, Singsen BH. Mixed connective tissue disease. In: *Arthritis and Allied Conditions* (McCarty DJ, Koopman WJ, eds.). Lea & Febiger: Philadelphia, 1993:1213–24.
29. Van Venrooij WJ, Sillekens PTG. Small nuclear RNA associated proteins: autoantigens in connective tissue diseases. *Clin Exp Rheumatol* 1989; **7**:635–45.
30. Van Venrooij WJ, Hoet R, Castrop J, Hageman B, Mattaj IW, Van de Putte LB. Anti-(U1) small RNA antibodies in anti-small nuclear ribonucleoprotein sera from patients with connective tissue diseases. *J Clin Invest* 1990; **86**:2154–60.
31. Rasmussen EK, Ullman S, Hoier-Madsen P, Sorensen SF, Halberg P. Clinical implications of ribonucleoprotein antibody. *Arch Dermatol* 1987; **123**:601–5.
32. Calderon J, Rodriguez-Valverde V, Sanchez Andrade S, Riestra JL, Gomez-Reyno J. Clinical profiles of patients with antibodies to nuclear ribonucleoprotein. *Clin Rheum* 1984; **3**:483–92.
33. Lázaro MA, Maldonado Cocco JA, Catoggio LJ, Babini SM, Messina OD, García Morteo O. Clinical and serologic characteristics of patients with overlap syndrome: is mixed connective tissue disease a distinct clinical entity? *Medicine* 1989; **68**:58–65.
34. Ter Borg EJ, Groen H, Horst G, Limburg PC, Wouda AA, Kallenberg CGM. Clinical associations of antiribonucleoprotein antibodies in

patients with systemic lupus erythematosus. *Semin Arthritis Rheum* 1990; **20**:164–73.
35. Konikoff F, Shoenfeld Y, Isenberg DA et al. Anti-RNP-antibodies in chronic liver diseases. *Clin Exp Rheumatol* 1987; **5**:359–61.
36. Gendi NST, Welsh KI, Van Venrooij WJ, Vancheeswaran R, Gilroy J, Black CM. HLA type as a predictor of mixed connective tissue disease differentiation. *Arthritis Rheum* 1995; **38:**259–66.
37. Pettersson I, Wang G, Smith EI, Wigzell H, Hedfors E, Horn J, Sharp GC. The use of immunoblotting and immunoprecipitation of (U) small nuclear ribonucleoproteins in the analysis of sera of patients with mixed connective tissue disease and systemic lupus erythematosus. A cross-sectional, longitudinal study. *Arthritis Rheum* 1986; **29**:986–96.
38. De Rooij DJRAM, Habets WJ, Van de Putte LBA, Hoet HM, Verbeek AL, Van Venrooij WJ. Use of recombinant RNP peptides 70K and A in an ELISA for measurement of antibodies in mixed connective tissue disease: a longitudinal follow-up of 18 patients. *Ann Rheum Dis* 1990; **49**:391–5.
39. Ter Borg EJ, Horst G, Limburg PC, Van Venrooij WJ, Kallenberg CGM. Changes in levels of antibodies against the 70 kDa and A polypeptides of The U1RNP complex in relation to exacerbations of systemic lupus erythematosus. *J Rheumatol* 1991; **18:**363–7.
40. Hoet RM, Koornneef I, De Rooij DJ, Van de Putte LB, Van Venrooij WJ. Changes in anti-U1 RNA antibody levels correlate with disease activity in patients with systemic lupus erythematosus overlap syndrome. *Arthritis Rheum* 1992; **35**:1202–10.
41. Habets WJ, De Rooij DJ, Salden MH, Verhagen AP, Van Eekelen CAG, Van de Putte LB, Van Venrooij WJ. Antibodies against distinct nuclear matrix components are characteristic for mixed connective tissue disease. *Clin Exp Immunol* 1983; **54**:265–76.
42. Netter HJ, Guldner HH, Szostecki C, Lakomek HJ, Will H. A recombinant auto-antigen derived from the human (U1) small nuclear RNP-specific 68-kd protein. *Arthritis Rheum* 1988; **31:**616–22.
43. Guldner HH, Netter HJ, Szostecki C, Lakomek HJ, Will HJ. Epitope mapping with a recombinant human 68-kDa (U1) ribonucleoprotein antigen reveals heterogeneous autoantibody profiles in human autoimmune sera. *J Immunol* 1988; **141**:469–75.
44. De Rooij DJ, Van de Putte LB, Habets WJ, Verbeek AL, Van Venrooij WJ. The use of immunoblotting to detect antibodies to nuclear and cytoplasmic antigens. *Scand J Rheumatol* 1988; **17**:353–64.
45. Reichlin M, Van Venrooij WJ. Autoantibodies to the URNP particles: relationship to clinical diagnosis and nephritis. *Clin Exp Immunol* 1991; **83**:286–90.
46. Craft J, Hardin J. Anti-snRNP antibodies. In: *Dubois' Lupus Erythematosus* (Wallace DJ, Hahn BH, eds.) 4th edn. Lea & Febiger: Philadelphia, 1993:216–24.
47. Ruuska P, Hämeenkorpi R, Forsberg S et al. Differences in HLA antigens between patients with mixed connective tissuedisease and systemic lupus erythematosus. *Ann Rheum Dis* 1992; **51**:52–5.
48. Black CM, Maddison PJ, Welsh KI, Bernstein R, Woodrow JC, Pereira RS. HLA and immunoglobulin allotypes in mixed connective tissue disease. *Artritis Rheum* 1988; **31**:131–4.
49. Hoffman RW, Rettenmaier LJ, Takeda Y et al. Human autoantibodies against the 70-kd polypeptide of U1 small nuclear RNP are associated with HLA-DR4 among connective tissue disease patients. *Arthritis Rheum* 1990; **33**:666–73.
50. Kaneoka H, Hsu K, Takeda Y, Sharp GC, Hoffman RW. Molecular genetic analysis of HLA-DR and HLA-DQ genes among anti-U1-70-kd autoantibody positive connective tissue disease patients. *Arthritis Rheum* 1992; **35**:83–94.
51. Hoffman RW, Sharp GC, Irvin WS, Anderson SK, Hewett JE, Pandey JP. Association of immunoglobulin Km and Gm allotypes with specific antinuclear antibodies and disease susceptibility among connective tissue disease patients. *Arthritis Rheum* 1991; **34**:453–8.
52. Genth E, Zarnowski H, Mierau R, Wohltmann D, Hartl PW. HLA-DR4 and Gm(1,3;5,21) are associated with U1-nRNP antibody positive connective tissue disease. *Ann Rheum Dis* 1987; **46**:189–96.
53. LeRoy EC, Maricq HR, Kahaleh MB. Undifferentiated connective tissue syndromes. *Arthritis Rheum* 1980; **23**:341–3.
54. Van den Hoogen FHJ, Boerbooms AMT, Spronk P, Bootsma H, de Rooij DJRAM, Kallenberg C, Van de Putte LBA. Mixed connective tissue disease – a farewell? *Br J Rheumatol* 1993; **32**:348–9.

10

Can the *Klebsiella* story in ankylosing spondylitis be laid to rest?

Bernard Amor and Antoine Toubert

INTRODUCTION

During the last 50 years an increasing number of infectious agents have been postulated to trigger reactive arthritis. Due to the frequency of overlap at the individual and family levels, between reactive arthritis and ankylosing spondylitis, plus the association of these two clinical entities with HLA-B27, the possible role of these infectious agents in ankylosing spondylitis has also been considered on the basis of clinical observations or epidemiological studies.

In contrast, the first step in the *Klebsiella pneumoniae* history in spondyloarthropathies was the result of an in vitro experiment. Thus, in 1973, Ebringer suggested that the extent of an immune response might be explained, to some degree, by the cross reactivity between the H2 complex of mice and foreign antigens, and assumed that the association of HLA and particular diseases could be explained by a similar mechanism. The serum of rabbits immunized with B27 lymphocytes from healthy donors was tested for reactivity with 32 microbes. The rabbit sera showed cross reactivity with three microbes: *Enterobacter aerogenes*, *K. pneumoniae* and *Yersinia enterocolitica*. Subsequently, monospecific anti-HLA-B27 sera compared with monospecific antisera against other HLA specificities on radiolabelled *K. pneumoniae* sonicated extracts were shown to give a stronger immune reaction (reviewed in references 1 and 2).

To support a role of *K. pneumoniae* in patients with ankylosing spondylitis two types of trials were developed: those exploring the clinical relevance of these experimental serological findings and those examining the relationship between *K. pneumoniae*, HLA-B27 and spondyloarthropathies.

CLINICAL STUDIES IN SUPPORT OF A ROLE OF *K. PNEUMONIAE* IN ANKYLOSING SPONDYLITIS

Isolation of *K. pneumoniae* in the faeces

Three studies have been published, with conflicting results. In the first, *K. pneumoniae* was isolated in 75% of patients with active ankylosing spondylitis, in 35% of those with probably active disease, in 20% of patients with inactive disease, in 16% of male controls, and in 8% of female controls.[3] These results were not confirmed by Warren and Brewerton 1978, cited in reference 4. Eastmond and colleagues[5] found faecal *K. aerogenes* (*K. pneumoniae* in the English nomenclature) in 27.1% of patients with ankylosing spondylitis and 34.1% of controls, and no significant association with spinal disease activity. They found an association with acute uveitis and active peripheral synovitis.

Since 1979, no other studies on the isolation of *K. pneumoniae* in the faeces have been published. Faecal flora contains thousands of bacterial species. Therefore, interpretation of the isolation of a nonpathogenic bacterial strain in asymptomatic patients is hazardous. Moreover, disease activity in ankylosing spondylitis is not easily defined.

IgA serum level in ankylosing spondylitis

Because IgA is the main immunoglobulin in mucosal tissue secretions, elevated IgA levels could be interpreted as a sign of the stimulation of the secretory immune system of the gastrointestinal tract due to mucosal infections.

A selective increase of serum IgA was first suggested in 1980 by Cowling, Ebringer and Ebringer,[6] and a persistent increase of the serum concentration of total IgA, secretory IgA, and some IgA subclasses in patients with ankylosing spondylitis has been described by others. A review of the literature concerning serum immunoglobulins in ankylosing spondylitis is not totally convincing of the specificity of an increase in IgA levels in patients with ankylosing spondylitis. Veys and van Laere[4] observed an increase in IgG, IgM, and IgA levels in cases of ankylosing spondylitis compared to normal subjects, but no statistically significant difference was found between IgM and IgA levels in patients with ankylosing spondylitis and those with rheumatoid arthritis (RA).

In the Cowling study, the selective increase of the IgA level was observed only during phases of active inflammatory disease. In this work and similar studies, serum immunoglobulins were measured in patients with ankylosing spondylitis during various phases of disease activity and compared to healthy controls. Two forms of bias may result from this methodology, as discussed by Dougados et al.[7] For example, 221 sera from 122 patients were selected randomly and compared to sera from healthy subjects. This choice meant that more than one serum sample was studied for some patients, and there was a possibility that the sera from the more active patients were stored more often, whereas only single serum samples were obtained from healthy subjects.

A second bias might occur if the results from the patients with ankylosing spondylitis are not compared with those with other inflammatory conditions, such as RA. It must be noted that an increased IgA level in ankylosing spondylitis patients is seen only when the erythrocyte sedimentation rate (ESR) exceeds 15 mm/h.

In an effort to avoid these two biases, the ESR and IgG, IgM, and IgA levels were measured[7] in single serum samples of 59 patients with ankylosing spondylitis who had only axial involvement, in 28 RA patients, and in 17 low back pain patients treated with nonsteroidal anti-inflammatory drugs, a good control, since ankylosing spondylitis and RA patients were both treated with these drugs. The ESR and IgA and IgG levels were statistically significantly increased in patients with ankylosing spondylitis and RA when compared to patients with low back pain. No statistically significant difference was observed for IgG or IgA levels in those with ankylosing spondylitis and RA. The ESR was elevated significantly in RA. The slight increase of the mean serum level of IgM in patients with RA was not statistically significantly different when compared with patients with ankylosing spondylitis and low back pain.

To discriminate between a selective or relative increase of IgA, the level of IgA expressed as a ratio with IgG was compared in the three groups, but no differences were observed. Nevertheless, in the longitudinal part of the study[7] conducted on 30 patients with ankylosing spondylitis who had both clinical and biological data collected at entry and after 3 and 6 months of follow-up, variations in the IgA level were found to correlate significally with a clinical index of activity. This correlation persisted after all the other variables were taken into account.

Subclasses of IgA in ankylosing spondylitis

Which subset of IgA is found in the sera of patients with ankylosing spondylitis? In normal sera, serum IgA is essentially 160-kDa monomers (mIgA), which are produced by the central immune system. A polymeric form (pIgA), mainly covalent dimers (330 kDa), which represents about 13% of serum IgA, is produced by the central immune system and by mucosa-associated lymphoid tissue. A subset of polymers of 400 kDa, similar to secretory IgA (sIgA), is present at a low level (11.5 mg/ml). The IgA1 subclass represents about 90% of the serum IgA, whereas the IgA1/IgA2 ratio varies from 0.7 to 2 in associated mucosal lymphoid tissue and secretions.[8]

In the study by Hocini et al[9] it was shown clearly that IgA in the sera of patients with ankylosing spondylitis were essentially mIgA, which are molecules produced by the central immune system, and that IgA1 was in the normal range in serum mIgA and pIgA. The serum concentrations were increased slightly, although nine patients had a concentration less than that of the normal serum pool. A weak but positive correlation ($P < 0.03$) between IgA and the ESR was found.

Antigenic specificities of IgA in ankylosing spondylitis

Mäki-Ikola and colleagues recently published three papers reporting the results of IgA antibody specificities in patients with ankylosing spondylitis. Sera of two groups of patients with ankylosing spondylitis (99 from Turku and 85 from Heinola in Finland) and of 102 healthy controls were used in the three studies. Antibodies to *K. pneumoniae*, *Escherichia coli*, and *Proteus mirabilis* and the lipopolysaccharides from *K. pneumoniae* and *E. coli* were first analysed by enzyme-linked immunosorbent assay (ELISA).[10] The investigators found an increased level of IgA class antibodies to *K. pneumoniae* in the peripheral and in the axial form of ankylosing spondylitis, and an increased level of IgM in patients with the peripheral form and of IgG in patients with the axial form of ankylosing spondylitis. However, specific IgA antibacterial antibodies were not restricted to *K. pneumoniae*. An increased level of IgA against *E. coli* and *P. mirabilis* was also found. The antibody level against the three bacteria had decreased in the sulphasalazine-compared to the placebo-treated patients by the 26th week of treatment.

From these data, the authors suggest that there is evidence of a role for *K. pneumoniae* in ankylosing spondylitis and that the immunoglobulin increase against *E. coli* and *P. mirabilis* can be explained by cross reactivity. Therefore, in the second study,[11] only IgA1 and IgA2 subclass-specific anti-*K. pneumoniae* antibodies in sera of patients with peripheral and axial types of ankylosing spondylitis were analysed. An increased level of both IgA subclasses was observed in the peripheral and the axial forms of ankylosing spondylitis compared to controls, but the differences in immunological findings between the two clinical aspects of ankylosing spondylitis suggested in the previous paper were not confirmed. Both IgA1 and IgA2 subclasses were involved in the disease. Serum IgA1 and IgA2 subclass antibody levels against *K. pneumoniae* bacteria were then compared for the presence or absence of extra-articular features such as iritis or enthesitis. The study was again focused on the *K. pneumoniae*-specific IgA antibody only. An extract of whole bacteria was used as the antigen in the ELISA. IgA1 and IgA2 levels in patients with or without iritis and with or without enthesitis were similar, but were statistically significantly higher than in healthy controls. The conclusion was that IgA1 and IgA2 antibody levels against the whole *K. pneumoniae* bacteria were both increased.[12]

The same group measured IgG, IgM, and IgA antibody levels against the same three enterobacteria in 25 patients with ankylosing spondylitis and 100 healthy controls, according to the endoscopic findings in ileocolonoscopy.[13] The patients with any type of endoscopic inflammatory findings in the gut usually had higher *Klebsiella* antibody levels than those without such inflammation. When compared to healthy controls, the ankylosing spondylitis patients with chronic gut inflammation had statistically significantly higher IgA and IgG class antibody levels against *K. pneumoniae*. In the patients without these inflammatory findings in the gut, these antibody levels were not increased. There were no differences seen in antibody levels against *E. coli* and *P. mirabilis* between the patients with or without these endoscopic findings and healthy controls. When the patients were grouped into axial and peripheral types of ankylosing spondylitis, the findings described above were seen only in the patients with the axial type of ankylosing spondylitis. The increased IgM and IgA anti-*K. pneumoniae* levels described in patients with the peripheral form of ankylosing spondylitis has not been confirmed.

Antibodies against *K. pneumoniae* in the small intestine of patients with ankylosing spondylitis

IgM, IgG, and IgA class antibodies against three different *K. pneumoniae* strains, and against *P. mirabilis* were measured by ELISA in jejunal perfusion fluids collected by a double balloon device in 19 patients with ankylosing spondylitis, 15 patients with RA, and 22 healthy controls.[14] The ankylosing spondylitis patients had significantly increased IgM, IgG, and IgA antibody levels against *K. pneumoniae* and had elevated IgM and IgA antibody levels against *E. coli* and *P. mirabilis*, when compared to healthy controls. When compared to patients with RA, the ankylosing spondylitis patients had higher levels of only IgA and IgG class antibodies against *K. pneumoniae*. The RA patients had higher IgM class antibody levels against all three enterobacteria studied, when compared to healthy controls. This study suggests an abnormal mucosal humoral immune response particularly to *K. pneumoniae* in ankylosing spondylitis patients.

From studies to date, it can be concluded that the clinical relevance of a role for *K. pneumoniae* in ankylosing spondylitis pathogenesis has not been clearly or consistantly established.

MIMICRY BETWEEN HLA-B27 AND *K. PNEUMONIAE* AT THE MOLECULAR LEVEL

Since the early 1980s much work has been devoted to the suspected role of *K. pneumoniae* in ankylosing spondylitis in terms of disease pathogenesis. Several hypotheses have been raised, leading to some passionate debates. These will now be considered dispassionately.

The 'Geczy' hypothesis

According to this hypothesis, an ankylosing spondylitis-specific modification of HLA-B27 might be due to an enteric organism and could be detected specifically by anti-*Klebsiella* sera raised in rabbits.[15] It was suggested that genes from a *Klebsiella* plasmid, carried or integrated in human cells after infection, could be responsible for this alteration. The difficulty encountered with this theory came from the inability of many laboratories, including our own, to reproduce the serological data initially reported or to detect the genetic element which could be responsible for such a modification.[16] A collaborative international exchange of material and data also failed to resolve the issue, and although this hypothesis was very attractive at its onset, it has not been supported further.

Identification of cross reactive epitopes between *K. pneumoniae* and HLA-B27

The 'molecular mimicry' hypothesis was described initially by Ebringer et al[17] who stated that epitopes may be shared between a self-protein, the HLA-B27 antigen, and bacterial antigens. Two main experimental approaches to confirm this have been undertaken.

The reactivity of *K. pneumoniae* membrane proteins with HLA-B27-specific monoclonal antibodies on Western blots was reported.[18] Proteins of two molecular weights were positive, one of 35 kDa and the other of 19 kDa. The 35-kDa group was shown to be the heat-modifiable OmpA protein from the outer membrane of most Gram-negative bacteria.[19] It is of interest that these antibodies react with a polymorphic immunodominant sequence of HLA-B27 at the end of the α-1 domain (residues 63–84).[20]

Another argument for mimicry was based upon sequence homologies between HLA-B27 and the protein sequences kept in databases. Schwimmbeck et al[21] reported a homology between the 72–77 sequence from the major B*2705 molecular subtype of HLA-B27 and residues 188–193 from *K. pneumoniae* nitrogenase (the 'QTDRED' sequence). Studies on the reactivity of patient's sera against synthetic peptides carrying the homologous sequence gave conflicting data.[23,24] This was probably due to the difficult interpretation of peptide ELISA assays with human sera. The reactivity of antisera raised against synthetic peptides with the QTDRED sequence on synovial tissues from patients with ankylosing spondylitis or reactive arthritis[24] could be a mere reflection of inflammation and increased class I expression.

On balance, we take the view that the sequence homology is of interest, but probably of little pathological significance.

'Molecular mimicry' at the T-cell level

The current knowledge of the structure of HLA-B27 and of its function in peptide presentation to T cells is at the origin of the so-called 'arthritogenic peptide' hypothesis. If correct, the disease should be mediated by cytotoxic T cells (CTLs) recognizing a bacterial or a self peptide in the context of HLA-B27. The description by Hermann et al of HLA-B27-restricted CTLs specific for *Yersinia* or *Salmonella* as well as autoreactive CTLs isolated from the synovial fluid of patients[25] supports this hypothesis. *K. pneumoniae*-reactive T cells have been investigated by the same group.[26] A quantitative reduction of *K. pneumoniae*-responsive T cells was found in the peripheral blood lymphocytes of patients with ankylosing spondylitis in comparison with healthy controls. Two CD4+ proliferative lines that recognized *K. pneumoniae* were isolated from the synovial fluid of a patient with active ankylosing spondylitis.

Another interesting observation was made by Scofield's group. By using the peptide-binding motif of HLA-B*2705 and sequence comparisons with Gram-negative bacteria, these authors showed that a sequence from HLA-B27 itself sharing similarities with bacteria-derived sequences (LRRYLENGK), could bind in vitro to HLA-B*2705.[27,28] Nothing is known about the natural presentation of this peptide in normal cells or from the synovial tissue of affected patients. The functional recognition of this peptide by CTLs also remains to be investigated. This work is, in our opinion, an attractive reappraisal of the 'molecular mimicry' hypothesis at the functional level.

CONCLUSIONS

From the studies carried out to date, some results are in favour of a role for *K. pneumoniae* in the pathogenesis of ankylosing spondylitis, for example the statistically significant increase of the specific anti-*K. pneumoniae* IgA level found when compared in healthy controls; the specificity of this finding is less clear when patients with ankylosing spondylitis were compared to patients with RA. However, the level of these antibodies has no part to play in the diagnosis, the follow-up, or the treatment of patients with ankylosing spondylitis.

Striking data favouring a link between *K. pneumoniae* and ankylosing spondylitis include the existence in a protein data bank of a Gram-negative enteric bacteria sequence shared with the peptide-binding motif of HLA-B27. One of these proteins is the *K. pneumoniae* nitrogenase molybdenum–iron protein.

The more recent research suggesting possible links between *K. pneumoniae* and ankylosing spondylitis can be summarized as follows. There is less efficient elimination of enterobacteria-derived peptide; or those enteric peptides that share sequences with B27 and that satisfy the requirements to bind B27 hold the potential for breaking tolerance to B27 sequences;[27] or, as suggested,[29] because of the large size of protein databases, it is easy to find five or six amino acid matches between unrelated proteins over-represented, because these protein motifs are functionally important.

The final words of the *Klebsiella* story have still to be written. If such a link was to be proved, physicians would await its impact on clinical practice with great interest.

REFERENCES

1. Ebringer A. La spondylarthrite ankylosante HLA B27 et la théorie de la tolérance croisée. *Rev Rhum* 1983; **50**:763–9.
2. Ebringer A. Ankylosing spondylitis is caused by *Klebsiella*. Evidence from immunogenetic, microbiologic, and serologic studies. *Rheum Dis Clin North Am* 1992; **18**:105–21.
3. Ebringer R, Cooke D, Cadwell DR, Cowling R, Ebringer A. Ankylosing spondylitis: *Klebsiella* and HLA B27. *Rheumatol Rehabil* 1977; **16**:190–6.
4. Veys E, van Laere M. Serum IgG, IgM and IgA levels in ankylosing spondylitis. *Ann Rheum Dis* 1983, **32**:493–6.
5. Eastmond CJ, Willshaw HE, Burgess P, Shinebaum R, Cooke EM, Wright V. Frequency of faecal *Klebsiella aerogenes* in patients with ankylosing spondylitis and controls with respect to individual features of the diseases. *Ann Rheum Dis* 1980; **3**:118–23.
6. Cowling P, Ebringer R, Ebringer A. Association of inflammation with raised serum IgA in ankylosing spondylitis. *Ann Rheum Dis* 1980; **39**:545–9.
7. Dougados M, Gaudouen Y, Blan M, Boumier P, Raichvarg D, Amor B. Vitesse de sédimentation globulaire et immunoglobulines sériques au cours de la pelvispondylite rhumatismale. *Rev Rhum Mal Osteoartic* 1987; **54**:273–8.
8. Mestecky J, Russel MW. IgA subclasses. In: subclasses in other immunoglobulins. *Monogr Allergy* 1986; **19**:277–301.
9. Hocini H, Iscaki S, Benlarache C, Vitalis L, Chevalier X, Larget-Pied B, Bouvet JP. Increased levels of serum IgA as IgA1 monomers in ankylosing spondylitis. *Ann Rheum Dis* 1992; **51**:790–2.
10. Mäki-Ikola O, Nissilä M, Lehtinen K, Leirisalo-Repo M, Toivanen P, Granfors K. Antibodies to *Klebsiella pneumoniae, Escherichia coli* and *Proteus mirabilis* in the sera of patients with axial and peripheral form of ankylosing spondylitis. *Br J Rheumatol* 1995; **34**:413–7.
11. Mäki-Ikola O, Nissilä M, Lehtinen K, Lerisalo-Repo M, Granfors K. IgA1 and IgA2 subclass antibodies against *Klebsiella pneumoniae* in the sera of patients with peripheral and axial types of ankylosing spondylitis. *Ann Rheum Dis* 1995; **54**:631–5.
12. Mäki-Ikola O, Lehtinen K, Granfors K. Similarly increased serum IgA1 and IgA2 subclass antibody levels against *Klebsiella pneumoniae* bacteria in ankylosing spondylitis patients with/without extra-articular features. *Br J Rheumatol* 1966; **35**:125–8.
13. Granfors K, Mäki-Ikola O, Leirisalo-Repo M. Association of gut inflammation with increased serum klebsiella specific antibody levels in patients with axial type of ankylosing spondylitis [abstract 1171]. *Arthritis Rheum* 1995; **38**:S348.
14. Granfors K, Mäki-Ikola O, Hällgren R, Enhanced local production of antibodies against *K. pneumoniae* in small intestine of patients with ankylosing spondylitis [abstract 1170]. *Arthritis Rheum* 1995; **38**:S348.
15. Geczy AF, Alexander K, Bashir HV, Edmonds JP, Upfold L, Sullivan J. HLA-B27, *Klebsiella* and ankylosing spondylitis: biological and chemical studies. *Immunol Rev* 1983; **70**:23–50.
16. Toubert A, Philippon A, Amor B. HLA-B27, ankylosing spondylitis and *K. pneumoniae*: toward a molecular approach. *J Rheumatol* 1987; **14**:391–3.
17. Ebringer A, Baines M, Childerstone M, Ghuloom M, Ptaszynska T. Etiopathogenesis of ankylosing spondylitis and the cross-tolerance hypothesis. In: *Advances in Inflammation Research*, vol 9. *The Spondylarthropathies* (Ziff M, Cohen SB, eds.). Raven Press: New York, 1985:101–28.
18. Van Bohemen CG, Grumet FC, Zanen HC. Identification of HLA-B27M1 and M2 cross-reactive antigens in *Klebsiella, Shigella* and *Yersinia. Immunology* 1984; **52**:607–9.
19. Zhang JJ, Hamachi M, Hamachi T, Zhao YP, Yu DTY. The bacterial outer membrane protein which reacts with anti-HLA-B27 antibodies is the OmpA protein. *J Immunol* 1989; **143**:2955–60.
20. Toubert A, Hamachi M, Raffoux C, Park MS, Yu DTY. Epitope mapping of an HLA-B27 monoclonal antibody that also reacts with a 35-kD bacterial outer-membrane protein. *Clin Exp Immunol* 1990; **82**:16–20.
21. Schwimmbeck PL, Yu DTY, Oldstone MBA. Autoantibodies to HLA-B27 in the sera of HLA-B27 patients with ankylosing spondylitis and Reiter's sydrome. Molecular mimicry with *Klebsiella pneumoniae* as potential mechanism of autoimmune disease. *J Exp Med* 1987; **166**:173–81.
22. Ewing C, Ebringer R, Tribbick G, Geysen M. Antibody activity in ankylosing spondylitis sera to two sites on HLA-B27.1 at the MHC groove region (within sequence 65–85), and to a

Klebsiella pneumoniae nitrogenase reductase peptide (within sequence 181–199). *J Exp Med* 1990; **171**:1635–47.

23. de Vries DD, Dekker-Saeys AJ, Gyodi E, Bohm U, Ivanyi P. Absence of autoantibodies to peptides shared by HLA-B27.5 and *Klebsiella pneumoniae* nitrogenase in serum samples from HLA-B27 positive patients with ankylosing spondylitis and Reiter's syndrome. *Ann Rheum Dis* 1992; **51**:783–9.
24. Husby G, Tsuchiya N, Schwimmbeck PL, Keat A, Pahle JA, Oldstone MBA, Williams RC. Cross-reactive epitope with *Klebsiella pneumoniae* nitrogenase in articular tissue of HLA-B27+ patients with ankylosing spondylitis. *Arthritis Rheum* 1989; **32**:437–45.
25. Hermann E, Yu DTY, Meyer zum Büschenfelde KH, Fleischer B. HLA-B27- restricted CD8 T cells derived from synovial fluids of patients with reactive arthritis and ankylosing spondylitis. *Lancet* 1993; **342**:646–50.
26. Hermann E, Sucké B, Droste U, Meyer zum Büschenfelde KH. *Klebsiella pneumoniae*-reactive T cells in blood and synovial fluid of patients with ankylosing spondylitis. *Arthritis Rheum* 1995; **38**:1277–82.
27. Scofield RH, Warren WL, Koelsch G, Harley JB. A hypothesis for the HLA-B27 immune dysregulation in spondyloarthropathy: contributions from enteric organisms, B27 structure, peptides bound by B27, and convergent evolution. *Proc Natl Acad Sci USA* 1993; **90**:9330–4.
28. Scofield RH, Kurien B, Gross T, Warren WL, Harley JB. HLA-B27 binding of peptide from its own sequence and similar peptides from bacteria: implications for spondyloarthropathies. *Lancet* 1995; **345**:1542–4.
29. Roudier C, Auger I, Roudier J. Molecular mimicry reflected through database screening: serendipity or survival strategy? *Immunol Today* 1996; **17**:357–8.

11

Does anything improve steroid-induced osteoporosis?

Roger Smith

INTRODUCTION

Amongst those interested in bone, the catastrophic skeletal effects of excessive naturally occurring and/or iatrogenic corticosteroids* are well known,[1–12] but elsewhere ignorance prevails.[13,14] Much is written about steroid-induced osteoporosis, but little is understood. Virtually every conference on osteoporosis has a session on corticosteroid-induced bone loss, but often this is a playground for cell biologists and cytokine enthusiasts rather than a forum for clinical care. Consequently those on glucocorticoids receive little help to maintain or restore their skeleton – often already attenuated by underlying disease – and then only when osteoporosis is established.[13] Although there is no a priori reason why patients on long-term steroids should have less competent care than those who are oestrogen deficient, this often seems to be the case. For instance a recent community study, which estimated that within the UK up to one-quarter of a million persons were taking oral steroids, showed that of 303 subjects on continuous oral steroids only 14% had received any treatment to prevent osteoporosis.[14]

This chapter examines measures to prevent corticosteroid bone loss as well as to correct it; it draws on the lessons of postmenopausal osteoporosis whilst recognizing that the skeletal effects of oestrogen deficiency and corticosteroid excess are different; it emphasizes the particular importance of prevention, since susceptible persons may lose bone within the first few weeks of starting steroids; and it provides some clinical advice to counteract steroid-induced bone loss. Recent reviews and extensive bibliographies are provided by Reid and Grey[6] and Lukert.[8]

*In this context the terms steroid, corticosteroid and glucocorticoid are used interchangeably.

IMPROVEMENT INCLUDES PREVENTION

The chapter title questions whether steroid-induced bone loss can be reversed (secondary prevention). In a perfect world this should never arise. Protection of the skeleton should begin at the same time as corticosteroid therapy (primary prevention), because the rate of steroid-induced bone loss gives no time for delay. This is all the more important because the skeleton may already be fragile due to underlying disease, such as rheumatoid arthritis, or oestrogen deficiency after the menopause. Clinical experience shows that some patients may indeed take steroids in large doses without significant skeletal harm, whereas others lose bone and fracture rapidly. However, it is not possible to predict who will fracture and who will not, although pretreatment densitometry is a very approximate guide, which makes prevention all the more important.

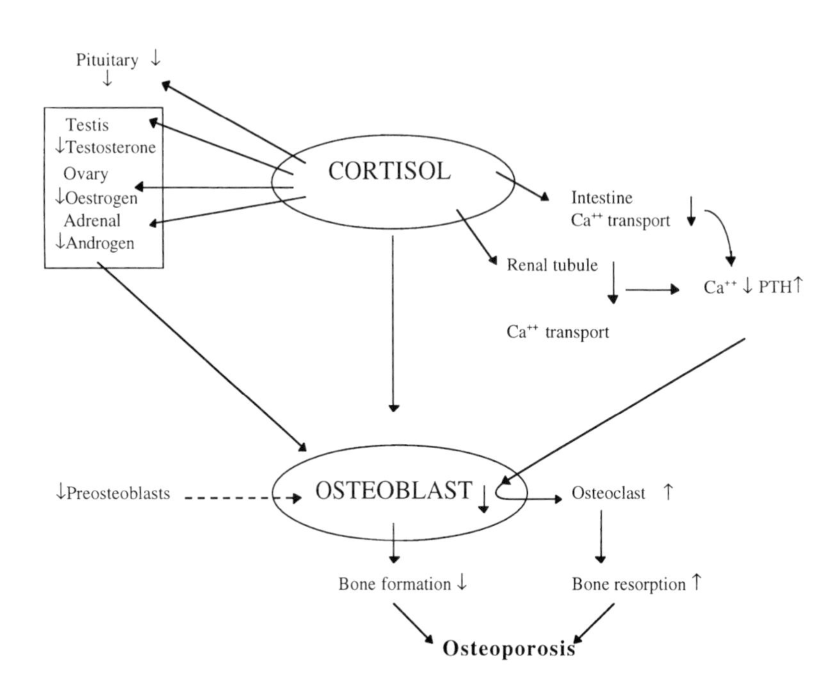

Figure 11.1 The multiple effects of corticosteroids on the skeleton, indicated by continuous arrows. The interrupted arrow indicates the origin of the osteoblast from the preosteoblast. PTH, parathyroid hormone.

BONE BIOLOGY

The effects of glucocorticoids on the skeleton are direct and indirect (Figure 11.1). Much evidence comes from work on animals and isolated cell systems;[8,11] some of it is conflicting and animal-specific, for instance, from mice and rats; and only a fraction can be applied to the human skeleton.

Bone cells

Glucocorticoids suppress the recruitment and activity of the osteoblasts.[8] This effect contrasts sharply with the increase in the rate of bone resorption and turnover in the perimenopause. Direct osteoblast suppression reduces the formation of new bone and causes generalized thinning of the bony trabeculae. The activity of osteoblasts is also reduced indirectly by sex hormone deficiency produced by the effect of cortisol on the gonads or adrenal directly or via the pituitary (Figure 11.1). Interestingly, in animal and human bone marrow cultures corticosteroids (notably dexamethasone) encourage the formation of osteoblasts, rather than adipocytes, from stromal cell precursors.[15,16]

There is current agreement that the major cellular effect of glucocorticoids falls on the osteoblast, but temporary and early bone resorption may also occur. This is thought to result largely from non-vitamin-D-related reduction in intestinal absorption and renal reabsorption of calcium, leading to an imperceptible fall in plasma calcium and an increase in parathyroid hormone (PTH) secretion (the evidence for and against this is discussed by Lukert[8] and Gulko and Mulloy[11]). Any effect of PTH on the osteoclast is probably mediated via the osteoblast.

Biochemistry

Since the effect of corticosteroids is primarily on bone formation, markers of this activity, particularly osteocalcin, show the most significant and rapid change.[17] There is a similar reduction in plasma procollagen type 1 C-terminal propeptide. No consistent changes occur in resorptive markers.[18]

Histology

Studies of bone histology have been very useful in understanding steroid-induced osteoporosis.[19,20] Suppression of bone formation leads to a reduction in mean wall thickness and a generalized lessening in trabecular width. In contrast to postmenopausal osteoporosis this suppression of formation (together with a variable increase in bone resorption) leads predominantly to a remodelling imbalance, which is more important than any increase in activation frequency of bone remodelling units. Trabeculae are (in general) not lost or perforated but merely thinned, so that their connectivity is retained and (in theory) the opportunity to reverse bone loss is greater than after the menopause. This is because the structure of trabecular bone (the type most affected by steroids) remains intact to serve as a potential template for new bone formation.

CLINICAL ASPECTS

General

The effects of glucocorticoids on the skeleton are set against the background of the underlying disease and depend on the dose and route of administration. Trabecular bones bear the brunt of steroid attack both in endogenous osteoporosis and in Cushing's syndrome; as a result the vertebrae are affected rapidly and severely and bones such as the ribs and pubic rami also show striking changes.[5] Apparently spontaneous fractures (which may be painless) occur at many sites and can be demonstrated by isotope bone scan. Radiographs confirm severe osteoporosis, including patchy loss of bone from the skull, and there is often striking hypertrophic callus at the site of fractures, including the end plates of wedged vertebrae. Osteonecrosis may contribute to vertebral fractures and to the collapse of femoral heads.

Underlying disease

Corticosteroids are given for many reasons: for example, to subdue sensitivity reactions, to avoid catastrophe (such as the impending blindness of temporal arteritis), to alleviate the effect of brain tumours, and to provide long-term control of chronic diseases, for which alternative treatments have proved to be ineffective – as in asthma or rheumatoid arthritis. In such chronic diseases, particularly rheumatoid arthritis and systemic lupus erythematosus, and in gastrointestinal problems such as Crohn's disease, there may be significant bone loss before corticosteroids are given, and hence less expectation of improvement. A more dramatic example of the effect of high-dose steroid therapy on a damaged skeleton is provided by the severe osteoporosis that can follow organ transplantation.[21]

Route and dose of corticosteroids

Corticosteroids induce bone loss roughly in proportion to the total amount given (derived from the daily dose and duration of therapy). The effects appear to be more marked for oral than inhaled preparations, but this may reflect the absorbed dosage. Since there is considerable individual variation in the skeletal response to corticosteroids, only general statements can be made about deleterious or harmless doses. Thus Lukert[8] states that the overall incidence of osteoporosis (defined as low bone mass or fracture, see below) in patients taking glucocorticosteroids for over 6 months is approximately 50%; further, she states that, in patients treated with large daily doses or inhaled steroids such as 1000–2000 μg of beclomethasone, the decrease in bone density is comparable to that seen in patients treated with oral prednisone 5–10 mg daily.[8] At three appendicular bone sites, elderly adults taking an average dose of 5 mg oral prednisone daily lost bone 2–3 times more rapidly than controls over an 8-year period.[12]

EXPECTATIONS FOR PREVENTION AND IMPROVEMENT

Cushing's syndrome

The most dramatic beneficial effects on the skeleton of reducing excess corticosteroids are

Table 11.1 Measures to prevent corticosteroid-induced osteoporosis

Proposals	Comments
Reduce corticosteroids	Keep dose low as possible
Use alternative drugs	Related to steroids, e.g. deflazacort. Immunosuppressives where appropriate
Specific measures	
Stimulate bone formation	
Exercise	To counteract myopathy as well as bone loss
Fluoride	Not widely used
Suppress bone resorption	
Hormone replacement	Oestrogen (plus progestogen) in women; testosterone in men
Bisphosphonates	Oral etidronate or alendronate. Possibly intravenous pamidronate
Calcium	Up to 1500 mg/day
Vitamin D	In physiological doses
Calcitonin	Not widely used
General lifestyle measures	
Avoid risk factors	Such as excessive alcohol, smoking, thinness
Additional calcium	As above
Appropriate exercise	
Good nutrition	To maintain muscle tissue

seen after the surgical correction of Cushing's syndrome.[22]

Relation to age

Whilst there is no reason to regard the adult skeleton as inert, the reversibility of corticosteroid-induced osteoporosis is best demonstrated in the growing skeleton, where the processes of bone modelling and remodelling are at their maximum.

Relation to cell biology

Since it is the osteoblast that is affected primarily by corticosteroids, potentially the most effective treatment to conserve the skeleton would be one that stimulates the osteoblasts. It is exactly in this area that our therapeutic armamentarium is most deficient.

OPTIONS FOR PREVENTION AND TREATMENT

In theory these are simple – reduce or stop corticosteroids or use alternative drugs; stimulate bone formation and reduce bone resorption. These should be combined with general lifestyle measures (Table 11.1). Apart from the first recommendation, much current advice derives from studies on postmenopausal osteoporosis.

Reduce corticosteroid dose

There is little to suggest that a threshold exists below which corticosteroids are harmless to the skeleton. However, 7.5 mg of prednisone or prednisolone daily is often regarded as physiological and therefore not likely to cause bone loss. In contrast, available evidence demonstrates increased bone loss at lower doses – especially in men and postmenopausal women;[8,12] and plasma osteocalcin levels may fall in patients given prednisone in doses as low as 2.5 mg daily.[23] Steroid replacement therapy for Addison's disease may also cause bone loss.[24]

Consequently the use of corticosteroids should be planned around the lowest effective dose, and with the avoidance of the systemic route wherever possible. Alternative methods of giving corticosteroids, such as on alternate days, show no skeletal advantages; inhaled corticosteroids can cause bone loss. Lukert[8] considers that even epidural corticosteroids given in sufficient dose could affect bone metabolism. Short courses of systemic large-dose corticosteroids (for instance methylprednisolone 1 g daily intravenously) in patients with rheumatoid arthritis may possibly avoid the deleterious effects of longer courses. For many years it has been suggested that some corticosteroids spare bone more than others with equal anti-inflammatory effects. One such is Deflazacort (an oxazolone derivative of prednisone); unfortunately this is not widely available, and evidence of its skeletal advantages compared with other steroids is sparse. One difficulty is the accurate assessment of its anti-inflammatory effect.[8]

Encourage bone formation

In practice there are only two ways of stimulating bone formation and osteoblastic activity. These are exercise and sodium fluoride.

Studies that measure the density of bone under mechanical stress demonstrate minor but often significant improvements induced by exercise at any age.[25] The benefits of exercise are more dramatic in the young skeleton, in which size increases as well as mass. The skeletal effects of exercise have not been formally demonstrated in patients on glucocorticoids, but the combination of bone loss and myopathy which these agents produce suggests that exercise should be included amongst the general lifestyle measures of the steroid-treated patient.

There is no doubt that fluoride stimulates the osteoblast to produce an excessive amount of bone. The demonstrated increase in spinal bone density is not paralleled by a reduction in fracture rates (which remain unchanged, or even increase, especially in the hip and peripheral skeleton). Current controversy – which continues – is concerned about whether there is a dose and preparation of sodium fluoride that increases bone density and reduces fracture rate. The therapeutic window between effectiveness and side-effects is very small; fluoride has many potential advantages, but its effects are unpredictable.[26,27] For these reasons it is not usually recommended in the management of steroid osteoporosis.

Reduce bone resorption

All the major available bone-sparing agents suppress the osteoclast. They reduce bone resorption and turnover and restore the balance between formation and resorption. These agents include hormone replacement therapy, bisphosphonates and calcitonin, together with calcium and vitamin D.

Antiresorptive agents have common effects on the skeleton which arise from the nature of the bone remodelling cycle.[28] There are numerous bone remodelling units throughout the skeleton. Reductions in bone resorption and bone turnover lead to a temporary increase in measured bone mineral density (BMD), as the osteoblasts in these units continue to fill the resorption lacunae. Since a bone remodelling cycle may take several months to complete, the increase in BMD is sustained for approximately the same length of time. In the second and subsequent years the increase may slow considerably or cease; or sometimes the loss of bone may resume at its previous rate. The outcome depends largely on the initial rate of bone turnover.[29] In practice this means that any antiresorptive agent will produce a temporary increase in bone density. Since the effectivenss of antiresorptive agents has often been assessed by short-term changes in bone density over 1–2 years without any measurements of fracture rate, their significance is in doubt. With these provisos, potentially the most effective agents for the prevention of corticosteroid bone loss are oestrogens (with progestogen where appropriate) and bisphosphonates. This has been demonstrated almost exclusively in postmenopausal women. In corticosteroid osteoporosis adequate long-term trials have yet to be done, and the differences in cell biology in the two types of osteoporosis should caution against too close an analogy.

Hormone replacement therapy

Hormone replacement therapy (HRT) prevents bone loss in postmenopausal women and those on HRT have a reduced rate of hip fracture.[30] Oestrogen also appears to have considerable cardiovascular benefits, reducing the risk of cardiovascular death by up to 50%. Postmenopausal women who have not had a hysterectomy need progestogen to counteract the endometrial hyperplasia and malignancy induced by oestrogen; the relative risk of breast cancer may be increased by approximately 1.3 to 1.4 after more than 10 years of oestrogen therapy. Also, three recent studies (reviewed in reference 31) have shown a slightly increased risk of venous thromboembolism in HRT users. These aspects have been discussed widely and provide a firm basis for HRT in hysterectomized women, but with current regimes the advantages of HRT for nonhysterectomized women are less clear.[32] Also, if we assume that a course of HRT is limited to 10 years (because of the possible increased risk of breast cancer thereafter), there is a difficulty in knowing which postmenopausal decade to choose. This is because there appears to be an increase in the rate of bone loss to early postmenopausal values as soon as HRT ceases. This means, for instance, that for a woman who has a decade of HRT from 50–60 years of age, the bone density after the age of 70 is no greater than if she had never had HRT.[33]

All these points are relevant to the oestrogen deficiency of women on corticosteroids. In postmenopausal women corticosteroid therapy is a strong additional indication for HRT, but the length of time for which HRT should be given is still controversial. It could be argued that the skeletal advantages of continuing HRT in the postmenopausal woman on corticosteroids for longer than 10 years outweigh the apparently increased risk of breast cancer.

Glucocorticoids reduce oestrogen levels before as well as after the menopause and HRT should therefore be given to premenopausal women with demonstrated oestrogen lack.

Bisphosphonates

Bisphosphonates are a family of simple inorganic compounds with a common P-C-P structure which block osteoclast-mediated bone resorption. Etidronate and the aminobisphosphonate alendronate have been shown to increase bone density and reduce the vertebral fracture rate in postmenopausal women, and possibly reduce the rate of nonvertebral fractures.[34,35] Another aminobisphosphonate (pamidronate) has been shown to be effective in glucocorticoid-induced osteoporosis, as assessed by significant benefits on bone density. Bisphosphonates are generally regarded as an alternative to HRT in postmenopausal women in whom HRT is inappropriate (e.g. if there is a personal or family history of breast cancer) or unacceptable. They are also potentially useful in young oestrogen-replete women or men on glucocorticoids. Although more information is necessary to establish their position in steroid osteoporosis, recent research (see below) strongly suggests that the bisphosphonates have a place both in the prevention and in the treatment of steroid-induced osteoporosis.[36]

Calcitonin

Calcitonin has a temporary beneficial effect on bone density, but there is little work on its long-term effects and none on fracture rate. Also, because of the significant side-effects (nausea, malaise, fever, etc) of systemic use, it is not widely used.[37] Nasal preparations are more acceptable, but their long-term skeletal effectiveness has yet to be proved.

Calcium and vitamin D

Current evidence demonstrates the beneficial effect of additional calcium on the skeleton at any age, especially where the prior intake is low, and also when associated with exercise.[38–40] It is proposed that this is due to a reduction in PTH-mediated bone resorption. Similarly, calcium plus vitamin D have been shown to reduce fracture rate in elderly women, despite rather small bone density advantages.[41] These skeletal aspects of additional calcium have been extensively reviewed.[42] Since glucocorticoids reduce calcium absorption (by a mechanism which may, however, be independent of vitamin D) there are good reasons for making sure that the patient on glucocorticoids takes sufficient (1000–1500 mg/day) calcium.

Corticosteroid osteoporosis in men

Corticosteroids reduce testosterone production and the circulating level should be measured; if this is found to be low, testosterone esters, rather than anabolic steroids, should be given by injection.[43]

General lifestyle measures

Luckily the prevention and treatment of bone loss and fracture do not rely entirely on a handful of bone-active drugs. Each patient on glucocorticoids should be treated as an individual; appropriate lifestyle measures are as important as in postmenopausal osteoporosis. In brief (Table 11.1) the corticosteroid dose should be reduced as far as possible compatible with the underlying disease; alternative drugs should be used where possible; the diet should contain sufficient protein, calcium, and vitamin D; mobility should be encouraged; smoking and excessive alcohol should be avoided; and (especially in young people) excessive thinness should be discouraged, since the deleterious effects of anorexia nervosa on the skeleton are well described.

The patient also needs advice on the prevention of fracture. Glucocorticoids produce proximal muscle weakness, which contributes to an increase in falls and subsequent fracture. The prevention of falls is an important part of the general advice given to people with osteoporosis; it includes measures to make the environment safe, to encourage appropriate exercise, to maintain mobility and to avoid the excessive use of prescribed and nonprescribed drugs.

MANAGEMENT OF STEROID-INDUCED OSTEOPOROSIS

What to use

Compared with the extensive work on postmenopausal osteoporosis there is relatively little on the management of steroid-induced bone loss. This has been reviewed recently by Lukert,[8] Sambrook and Jones[9] and Sambrook.[44] Lukert[8] finds that with HRT in postmenopausal women who are also on glucocorticoids, the expected skeletal advantage is demonstrated; the use of 1α-hydroxylated metabolites or vitamin D is regarded by her as controversial until more information is available; the studies of calcitonin in patients on glucocorticoids have been too short to be of significance. With bisphosphonates several studies exist that have involved etidronate and pamidronate. Again these studies are considered to be too short to be clinically significant and their effectivenss is judged solely from short-term changes in bone density. Sambrook and Jones[9] came to largely similar conclusions after reviewing the available clinical trials with different therapeutic agents and classifying them according to the primary prevention (with steroids not having previously been given) or treatment (secondary prevention) of established bone loss. In their view most of the studies reviewed were inadequate and all were short; additionally they were all judged by short-term changes in bone density. However, Sambrook[44] later concluded that either calcitriol or the bisphosphonate etidronate should be considered in the primary prevention of corticosteroid-induced bone loss. Whilst the desirability of fracture studies is accepted widely, it is very difficult to study the number of patients required to establish a significant change in vertebral fracture rate within a reasonable time.

Two recent reports serve to emphasize the continuing difficulty in assessment of regimes for the prevention and treatment of steroid-induced osteoporosis.[45,46] Diamond et al[42] gave 15 postmenopausal women cyclical etidronate, ergocalciferol and calcium at the same time as they began glucocorticoid treatment. The nonrandom 'historical' control group consisted of 11 postmenopausal women with established glucocorticoid osteoporosis on calcium supplements only. In the women on etidronate plus vitamin D, bone loss was prevented. Clearly there are many uncertainties about such a study, which include the problem of inadequate controls and the question of whether the bone-sparing effect was due to etidronate or vitamin D. Rizzoli et al[46] described the effect of sodium monofluorophosphate on bone density in 48 men and women with established corticosteroid-induced osteoporosis. In this treatment study they showed the expected increase in spinal BMD, without any changes in the femur BMD or any troublesome side-effects. The study was partly random and partly open and the changes were compared with a group of patients (two men, 15 women) with idiopathic osteoporosis.

Recently published work emphasizes the possibility of primary prevention of steroid-induced bone loss and demonstrates that when the bisphosphonate pamidronate is given virtually at the same time as corticosteroid therapy is begun it will prevent significant bone loss over the following 2 years, in contrast to a group given pamidronate 3 months after corticosteroids are started.[47] This protection of the skeleton mirrors the beneficial effect of cyclical etidronate in established steroid osteoporosis.[48] Another recent study in established steroid osteoporosis demonstrates the beneficial effect of injected testosterone esters on lumbar BMD in men.[49] However, Adachi and colleagues[50] found no convincing evidence that long-term native vitamin D (50 000 units weekly) and calcium (1000 mg daily) had any skeletal benefit for those on long-term corticosteroids.

Therefore, good clinical trials remain remarkably few. Polypharmacy, short-term measurement, and lack of appropriate controls make the results difficult to interpret. Virtually any agent expected to be beneficial from its known effects on bone biology can be shown to be so assessed by short-term changes in bone density; what this means with regard to fracture can only be dimly surmised!

Whom to treat

Few authors deal specifically with this question. By implication some consider that for all those who start on a course of glucocorticoids which is likely to be long term (this is difficult to define, but more than a few weeks would be appropriate) care of the skeleton should be planned from the start[8] (Figure 11.2). Clearly this is not common practice. Others[51] restrict themselves to the management of patients with established osteoporosis (BMD lower than 2.5 standard deviations (SD) below peak bone mass – T score) or with an age-matched BMD (Z score) lower than 1 SD below the mean, or patients about to embark on a course of corticosteroid therapy likely to last for more than 6 months with a mean daily dose of more than 15 mg of prednisone (Figure 11.3). This latter scheme means that those whose initial bone density does not come within these definitions or who will be on lesser doses of steroids are disregarded, except for advice about general measures.[51]

There is an important difference in these proposals. In the first (Figure 11.2), bone-sparing

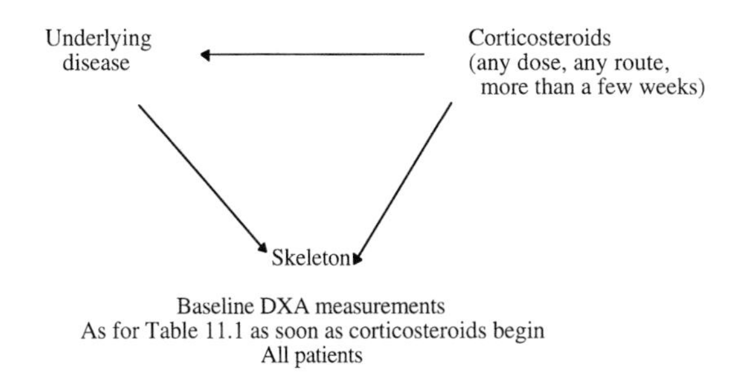

Figure 11.2 Scheme for the primary prevention of steroid-induced osteoporosis. This diagram emphasizes that the skeleton is affected by both the underlying diseases and the corticosteroid therapy. All patients should begin bone-sparing regimes when corticosteroids are started.

therapy is begun at the same time as corticosteroids, irrespective of bone density, steroid dose, and likely duration of steroid therapy, whereas in the second (Figure 11.3) bone-sparing drugs are given only if the skeleton is already osteoporotic or likely to become so due to excessive steroids.

Thus the proposals in Figure 11.2 differ from those of Eastell et al[51] (Figure 11.3), since the therapeutic decisions do not rely so much on the bone mineral density results. It is recommended here that all patients who are likely to have long-term (defined as more than a few weeks) steroid therapy should receive advice about the maintenance of their skeleton with measures for primary prevention of bone loss, irrespective of their measured bone density. (Nevertheless, the pretreatment BMD provides important information about prognosis and a baseline for any further measurements that may be considered to be necessary.) There certainly seems little logic in treating only those with densitometric osteoporosis (T score 2.5 SD or more below peak bone mass, or age-matched Z score 1 SD or more below the mean), and disregarding others (apart from using general measures), only to treat them if they lose sufficient bone to be defined as osteoporotic a year later. This represents the loss of an opportunity to prevent iatrogenic bone loss and, presumably, fracture.

CURRENT CLINICAL PRACTICE

Two recent studies emphasize the widespread use of corticosteroids in hospital and in the community, and hence the considerable

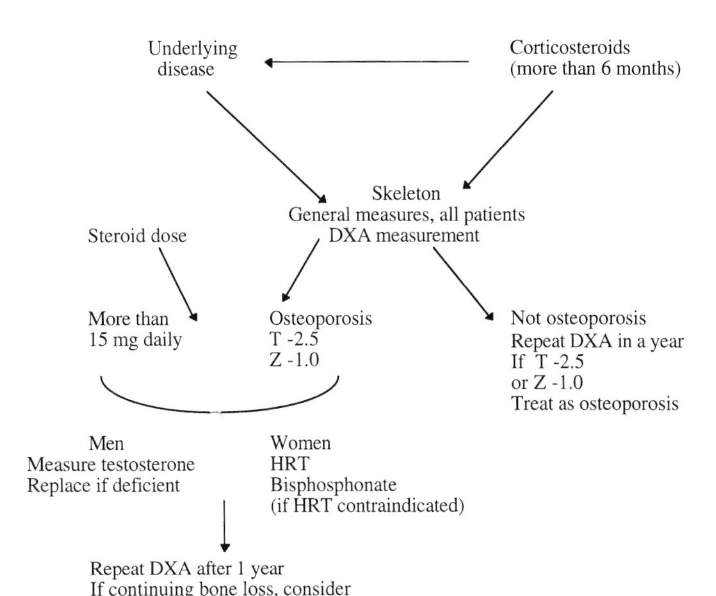

Figure 11.3 Scheme for the management of steroid-induced osteoporosis (partly based on Eastell[51]). Bone-sparing regimes are limited to those with densitometric osteoporosis or likely to be on prolonged (more than 6 months) high-dose (more than 15 mg prednisolone daily) regimes.

number of patients at risk from secondary osteoporosis. In a teaching hospital in Scotland 214 patients had corticosteroids prescribed over a 3-month period, but only 12 of them received any form of osteoporosis prophylaxis; also in postmenopausal women on corticosteroids (who are at particular skeletal risk) only 6% had any prophylaxis.[13] Similarly in a study (previously referred to) in eight large general practices around Nottingham,[14] 0.46% were currently on continuous oral corticosteroid therapy and of 303 patients only 41 (mostly women) had received treatment for the prevention of osteoporosis in the preceding 4 years.

This study suggested that, within the UK, some quarter of a million people are likely to be taking oral corticosteroids. As these patients are clearly identifiable (by reason of their prescription) and have a significant (perhaps fourfold) increase in fracture rate, much more needs to be done.

CONCLUSIONS

There is no doubt about the severity and extent of steroid-induced osteoporosis, but this is largely disregarded by clinicians. Current management is largely based on the evidence from postmenopausal osteoporosis. It is recommended that all those who begin steroids should be given advice about protection of their skeleton and should begin bone-sparing treatment. Assessment should include measurement of bone mineral density, but the results should not exclude any patient from advice.

Some current evidence suggests that early steroid-induced bone loss may be prevented (primary prevention) and that established corticosteroid osteoporosis can be ameliorated (secondary prevention), but an associated reduction in fracture rate has not been demonstrated. Detailed recommendations for the prevention and treatment of glucocorticoid osteoporosis have been published by the American College of Rheumatology Task Force on Osteoporosis.[52] In general, these agree with the news expressed here, particularly with regard to the importance of measuring BMD and starting measures to present bone loss as soon as corticosteroid therapy has begun.

REFERENCES

1. Gennari C, Civitelli R. Glucocorticoid osteoporosis. *Clin Rheum Dis* 1986; **12**:637–54.
2. Reid IR. Steroid osteoporosis. *Calcif Tiss Int* 1989; **45**:63–7.
3. Reid IR, Pathogenesis and treatment of steroid osteoporosis. *Clin Endocrinol* 1989; **30**:83–103.
4. Lukert BP, Raisz LG. Glucocorticoid-induced osteoporosis: Pathogenesis and management. *Ann Med* 1990; **112**:353–64.
5. Smith R. Corticosteroids and osteoporosis. *Thorax* 1990; **45**:573–8.
6. Reid IR, Grey AB. Corticosteroid osteoporosis. *Baillière's Clin Rheum* 1993; **7**:573–87.
7. Prince RL. Corticosteroid hormones. In: *Metabolic Bone and Stone Disease*, 3rd edn (Nordin BEC, Need AG, Morris HA, eds.). Churchill Livingstone: Edinburgh, 1993:43–56.
8. Lukert B. Glucocorticoid-induced osteoporosis. In: *Osteoporosis*, 1st edn (Marcus R, Feldman D, Kelsey J, eds.). Academic Press: New York, 1996:801–20.
9. Sambrook PN, Jones G. Corticosteroid osteoporosis. *Br J Rheum* 1995; **34**:8–12.
10. Compston JE. Glucocorticoid-induced osteoporosis In: *Current Research in Osteoporosis and Bone Mineral Measurement IV*. British Institute of Radiology: London, 1996:34–5.
11. Gulko PS, Mulloy AL. Glucocorticoid-induced osteoporosis: Pathogenesis, prevention and treatment. *Clin Exp Rheumatol* 1996; **14**:199–206.
12. Saito JK, Davis JW, Washnich RD, Ross PD. Users of low dose corticosteroids have increased bone loss rates: a longitudinal study. *Calcif Tiss Int* 1995; **57**:115–19.
13. Peat ID, Healy S, Reid DM, Ralston SH. Steroid-induced osteoporosis: an opportunity for prevention? *Ann Rheum Dis* 1995; **54**:66–8.
14. Walsh LJ, Wong CA, Pringle M, Tattersfield AE.

Use of oral corticosteroids in the community and prevention of secondary osteoporosis: a cross sectional study. *Br Med J* 1996; **313**:44–6.

15. LeBoy PS, Beresford JN, Devlin C, Owen ME. Dexamethasone induction of osteoblast mRNAs in rat marrow stromal cell cultures. *J Cell Physiol* 1991; **146**:370–8.
16. Beresford JN, Joyner CJ, Devlin C, Triffitt JT. The effects of dexamethasone and 1,25-dihydroxyvitamin D_3 on osteogenic differentiation of human marrow stromal cells in vitro. *Arch Oral Biol* 1994; **39**:941–7.
17. Peretz A, Praet J-P, Bosson D, Rosenberg S, Bourdoux P. Serum osteocalcin in the assessment of corticosteroid-induced osteoporosis. Effect of long term corticosteroid treatment. *J Rheumatol* 1989; **16**:363–7.
18. Prummel WF, Wiersinga WM, Kips P, Sanders GTB, Sauerwein HP. The course of biochemical parameters of bone turnover during treatment with corticosteroids. *J Clin Endocrinol Metab* 1991; **72**:382–6.
19. Aaron JE, Francis RM, Peacock M, Makins NE. Contrasting anatomy of idiopathic and corticosteroid-induced osteoporosis. *Clin Orthop Relat Res* 1989; **243**:294–305.
20. Dempster DW. Bone histomorphometry in glucocorticoid-induced osteoporosis. *J Bone Miner Res* 1989; **4**:137–41.
21. Sambrook PN, Kelly J, Fontan D, Bguyen T, Keogh A, MacDonald P, Sprat P, Freund J, Eisman JA. Mechanisms of rapid bone loss following organ transplantation. *Osteoporosis Int* 1994; **4**:273–6.
22. Pocock NA, Eisman JA, Dunstan CR, Evans RA, Thomas DH, Hug NL. Recovery from steroid-induced osteoporosis. *Ann Int Med* 1987; **107**:319–23.
23. Lukert BP, Higgins JC, Stoskopf MM. Serum osteocalcin is increased in patients with hyperthyroidism and decreased in patients receiving glucocorticoids. *J Clin Endocrinol Metab* 1986; **62**:1056–8.
24. Zeilissen PMJ, Croughs RJM, Van Rink PP, Raymakers JA. Effect of glucocorticoid therapy on bone mineral density in patients with Addison's disease. *Ann Int Med* 1994; **12**:207–10.
25. Snow CM, Matkin CC, Shaw JM. Physical activity and the risk for osteoporosis. In: *Osteoporosis*, (Marcus R, Feldman D, Kelsey J, eds.). Academic Press: New York, 1996:511–28.
26. Riggs BL, Hodgson SF, O'Fallon WM et al. Effect of fluoride treatment on the fracture rate in postmenopausal women with osteoporosis. *N Engl J Med* 1990; **322**:822–909.
27. Pak CYC, Sakhee K, Adams-Huet B et al. Treatment of postmenopausal osteoporosis with slow release sodium fluoride. *Ann Int Med* 1995; **123**:401–8.
28. Dempster DW, Lindsay R. Pathogenesis of osteoporosis. *Lancet* 1993; **341**:797–801.
29. Riggs BL, Melton LJ. The prevention and treatment of osteoporosis. *N Engl J Med* 1992; **327**:620–7.
30. Gallagher JC. Estrogen: prevention and treatment of osteoporosis. In: *Osteoporosis* (Marcus R, Feldman D, Kelsey J, eds.). Academic Press: New York, 1996:1191–208.
31. Vandenbrouke JP, Helmerhorst FM. Risk of venous thrombosis with hormone replacement therapy. *Lancet* 1996; **348**:972.
32. Grady D, Rubin SM, Pettiti DB, Fox CS, Black D, Ettinger D, Ernster VL, Cummings SR. Hormone replacement therapy to prevent disease and prolong life in postmenopausal women. *Ann Int Med* 1992; **117**:1016–37.
33. Smith R. Prevention and treatment of osteoporosis; common sense and science coincide. *J Bone Joint Surg* 1994; **76B**:345–7.
34. Marcus R. Cyclic etidronate; has the rose lost its bloom? *Am J Med* 1993; **95**:555–6.
35. Liberman VA, Weiss SR, Broll J et al. Effect of alendronate on bone mineral density and incidence of fractures in postmenopausal osteoporosis. *N Engl J Med* 1995; **333**:1437–43.
36. Gallacher SJ. Bisphosphonates. Role in treatment of corticosteroid-induced osteoporosis. *Clin Immunother* 1996; **6**:154–62.
37. Stock JL. Drug therapy. In: *Osteoporosis: Diagnostic and Therapeutic Principles* (Rosen CJ, ed.). Humana Press: New Jersey, 1996:173–87.
38. Dawson-Hughes B, Dallal GE, Krall EA, Sadowski L, Sahyoun N, Tannenbaum S. A placebo trial of the effect of calcium supplements on bone density in post-menopausal women. *N Engl J Med* 1990; **323**:878–83.
39. Prince RL, Smith M, Dick IM, Price RI, Webb PG, Henderson NK, Harris MM. Prevention of postmenopausal osteoporosis. A comparative study of exercise, calcium supplementation and hormone replacement therapy. *N Engl J Med* 1991; **325**:1189–95.
40. Dawson-Hughes B. The role of calcium in the treatment of osteoporosis. In: *Osteoporosis* (Marcus R, Feldman D, Kelsey J, eds.). Academic Press: New York, 1996:1159–68.

41. Chapuy MC, Arlot ME, Duboeuf F, Brun J, Crouzet S, Arnaud S, Delmas PD, Meunier PJ. Vitamin D3 and calcium to prevent hip fracture in elderly women. *N Engl J Med* 1992; **327**:1637–42.
42. Heaney RP. Thinking straight about calcium. *N Engl J Med* 1993; **328**:503–5.
43. Christiansen C. Androgens and androgenic progestins. In: *Osteoporosis* (Marcus R, Feldman D, Kelsey J, eds.). Academic Press: New York, 1996:1279–92.
44. Sambrook PN. Calcium and vitamin D therapy in corticosteroid bone loss; what is the evidence. *J Rheumatol* 1996; **23**:963–4.
45. Diamond T, McGuigan L, Barbagall S, Bryant C. Cyclical etidronate plus ergocalciferol prevents glucocorticoid-induced bone loss in post-menopausal women. *Am J Med* 1995; **98**:459–63.
46. Rizzoli R, Chevalley T, Slosman DO, Bonjour J-P. Sodium monofluorophosphate increases bone mineral density in patients with corticosteroid-induced osteoporosis. *Osteoporosis Int* 1995; **5**:39–46.
47. Wimalawansa S. Pre-stabilization of the skeleton with pamidronate can prevent steroid-induced osteoporosis. *J Bone Miner Res* 1996; **11** (Suppl): S498.
48. Adachi JD, Cranney A, Goldsmith CH et al. Intermittent cyclic therapy with etidronate in the prevention of corticosteroid-induced bone loss. *J Rheumatol* 1994; **21**:1922–26.
49. Reid IR, Wattie DJ, Evans MC, Stapleton JP. Testosterone therapy in glucocorticoid-treated men. *Arch Int Med* 1996; **156**:1173–7.
50. Adachi JD, Bensen WG, Bianchi F et al. Vitamin D and calcium in the prevention of corticosteroid-induced osteoporosis: A 3 years follow-up. *J Rheumatol* 1996; **23**:995–1000.
51. Eastell R. Management of corticosteroid-induced osteoporosis. *J Int Med* 1995; **237**:439–47.
52. American College of Rheumatology Task Force on Osteoporosis. Recommendations for the prevention and treatment of glucocorticoid – induced osteoporosis. *Arthritis Rheum* 1996; **39**:1791–801.

12

The classification and nomenclature of idiopathic peripheral arthritis in children

James T Cassidy

In this chapter the nomenclature of idiopathic peripheral arthritis in children is examined and the central question asked – have international disputes about the names given to chronic arthritis in children achieved anything? These names principally revolve around use of the terms *juvenile rheumatoid arthritis* (JRA), *juvenile chronic arthritis* (JCA), and *juvenile arthritis* (JA). These designations have been applied in part or whole to a number of closely related rheumatic diseases of children or a series of host responses that are characterized predominantly by idiopathic peripheral arthritis.[1] Current scientific evidence implicates an immunoinflammatory pathogenesis that may be activated by contact with an external antigen or antigens, in a host with a specific immunogenetic predisposition. Unfortunately, a sometimes heated controversy has swirled around these terms internationally for some 25 years, unresolved, and adamantly perpetuated.[2–7] Otherwise, this chapter would be unnecessary, and unanimity of outlook would descend upon the small paediatric rheumatology community. It is this hope, approached as nearly as possible, that should be our goal in once again reviewing these matters.

CURRENT NOMENCLATURE AND CLASSIFICATION CRITERIA

The term JRA was chosen by the first American College of Rheumatology (ACR) criteria subcommittee in 1963, as it had become well established in scientific usage in North America.[8] The first set of classification criteria were published in 1972 based upon a retrospective examination of data from nine clinics, and a subsequent prospective evaluation of the Delphic or nominal group definitions in 16 clinics.[9] These criteria were extended in 1977 to define the three principal types of onset based upon a constellation of clinical signs and symptoms present during the first 6 months of the illness (Table 12.1).[10] Finally

Table 12.1 Criteria for the classification of juvenile rheumatoid arthritis

1. Age at onset < 16 years
2. Arthrtitis (swelling or effusion, or presence of two or more of the following signs: limitation of range of motion, tenderness or pain on motion, and increased heat) in one or more joints
3. Duration of disease 6 weeks or longer
4. Onset type defined by type or disease in first 6 months:
   (a) Polyarthritis: ≥ 5 inflamed joints
   (b) Oligoarthritis: $\leqslant 4$ inflamed joints
   (c) Systemic: arthritis with intermittent fever
5. Exclusion of other forms of juvenile arthritis

Modified from reference 11.

Table 12.2 Outcome of juvenile rheumatoid arthritis by onset type. Numbers of children in parentheses

Onset type	Course subtype	Profile	Outcome
Polyarthritis (78)	RF seropositive (16)	Female Older age Hand/wrist Erosions Nodules Unremitting	Poor
	ANA seropositive (38)	Female	Good
	Seronegative (24)		Variable
Oligoarthritis (121)	ANA seropositive (66)	Female Young age Chronic uveitis	Excellent (except eyes)
	RF seropositive (8)	Polyarthritis Erosions Unremitting	Poor
	HLA B27-positive (12)	Male Older age	Good
	Seronegative (35)		Good
Systemic disease (51)	Oligoarthritis (30)		Good
	Polyarthritis (21)	Erosions	Poor

RF, rheumatoid factor; ANA, antinuclear antibody; HLA, human leukocyte antigen. From reference 12.

in 1986[11] and 1989,[12] course subtypes derived from the onset types were defined by cluster analysis of large cohorts of children (250 and 461) that had been prospectively studied at the University of Cincinnati (Table 12.2). Since then, these are the only criteria that have been studied by rigorously defined statistical evaluations to have face and content validity and to provide expectations of outcome based upon a 5-year course of the disease.

A European League Against Rheumatism (EULAR) Conference on *The Care of Rheumatic Children*, held in Oslo in 1977, proposed the term JCA for these heterogeneous disorders (Table 12.3).[13] The same three onset types were selected as in the ACR criteria and definitions of age of onset and duration of disease were similar. Although it was not possible to test these criteria prospectively at that time, the onset types were subsequently evaluated by Prieur et al.[14] Juvenile ankylosing spondylitis and juvenile psoriatic arthritis were included in these criteria. More recently, attempts have been made to establish sets of criteria for spondylitis and psoriatic arthritis, although their early diagnosis is still acknowledged to be difficult in many children.[15,16]

The classification criteria for JRA and JCA are compared in Table 12.4. They include a clinical definition of objective arthritis, age of onset,

Table 12.3 Criteria for the classification of juvenile chronic arthritis

1. Age at onset < 16 years
2. Arthritis in one or more joints
3. Duration of disease 3 months or longer
4. Type defined by characteristics at onset:
   - Pauciarticular: < 5 joints
   - Polyarticular: > 4 joints, rheumatoid factor negative
   - Juvenile rheumatoid arthritis: > 4 joints, rheumatoid factor positive
   - Systemic arthritis with characteristic fever and rash
   - Juvenile ankylosing spondylitis
   - Juvenile psoriatic arthritis
   - Arthritis of inflammatory bowel disease
5. Exclusion of other forms of juvenile arthritis

Modified from European League Against Rheumatism (EULAR) Bulletin 4, *Nomenclature and Classification of Arthritis in Children.* Basel, National Zeitung AG, 1977.

Table 12.4 Comparison of ACR and EULAR criteria for idiopathic peripheral arthritis in children

	ACR (JRA)	EULAR (JCA)
Age at onset (years)	< 16	< 16
Definition of arthritis	Yes	No
Duration of disease	⩾ 6 weeks	⩾ 3 months
Onset types	3	3
Course subtypes	9	—
Inclusion of JAS, psoriatic arthritis, and the arthritis of IBD	No	Yes
Exclusion of other forms of arthritis	Yes	Yes

JRA, juvenile rheumatoid arthritis; JCA, juvenile chronic arthritis; JAS, juvenile ankylosing spondylitis; IBD, inflammatory bowel disease.

duration of disease necessary for inclusion, and the three principal types of onset. Both sets of criteria indicate the need to exclude, where possible, all of the other rheumatic diseases of childhood. Each suffers equally, however, from the disadvantage of the lack of tested criteria for most of these other rheumatic diseases. Indeed, with few exceptions for the myriad disorders of children who present with peripheral arthritis, either criteria have not been subjected to prospective analyses, or classifications have been based upon modifications of adult criteria.

The EULAR criteria were derived from an extensive experience of diagnosing and treating children with these diseases at Taplow, and publications by Ansell and Bywaters in 1959,[17] 1962,[18] 1968,[19] and 1976.[20] The English criteria for juvenile chronic polyarthritis originally included closely related diseases such as systemic lupus erythematosus, and additional diagnostic procedures such as the requirement for a synovial biopsy in children with monarticular arthritis. In this classification, the term JRA was reserved for children with polyarthritis who were persistently seropositive for rheumatoid factors.

In fact, at this point a clarification of the objective of this discussion is in order; that is, to point out that these controversies have principally surrounded the *names* that have been in use, rather than the *criteria* defining the subsets identified by these names. As will be discussed, classification criteria have continued to evolve for these diseases and recently a new programme of evaluation was proposed by a select committee of the International League Against Rheumatism (ILAR).[21]

CRITERIA DEFINITIONS

It should be noted that there was no biological justification for selecting an age of 16 years at onset as an exclusion from these classifications. This criterion was originally chosen by the ACR subcommittee because this age represented a territorial distinction between children likely to be referred to paediatric clinics vs those who might initially be seen by specialists in internal medicine. With current changes in patterns of referral and health care, it seems likely that this age should be reconsidered in the development of new criteria.

Although 6 weeks of duration of disease was selected from the initial prospective analyses of the ACR subcommittee for a firm diagnosis, the EULAR criteria and those from Norway,[22] Sweden,[23] and Finland[24] have chosen a longer–period of 3 months. As this time of documentation of objective arthritis is an extremely important criterion for exclusion, this matter should be carefully re-examined in tentative sets of criteria along with the time required for establishment of the type of onset of disease, e.g. 6 months.

In addition, although it was possible in the Cincinnati data to identify course subtypes within the first 5 years of disease,[11] the ACR subcommittee did not examine whether a shorter interval would suffice. Unfortunately, data already exist to indicate that the risk of developing certain complications of these diseases, e.g. chronic anterior uveitis, is probably never limited by time after onset, although the vast majority of cases still occur within a defined period of time, in this case approximately 7 years.[25] Finally, it would be well to recall that the types of outcomes defined for these onset types and course subtypes are not restricted to any specific period of years, but are cumulative events based upon a variety of medical and nonmedical factors, such as family structure, socioeconomic status, compliance, availability of resources, and responses to treatment.

PURPOSES OF CLASSIFICATION CRITERIA

Classification criteria for the rheumatic diseases of children characterized by arthritis of the appendicular skeleton were developed because each of these clinical disorders lacked *a single distinguishing or diagnostic feature* that separated that entity from all similar types of arthritis in children, and from the larger universe of healthy children without these diseases. The ACR criteria were derived from combinations of clinical and laboratory manifestations that were selected from large prospectively assembled data sets by segregation analysis and identification of clusters of signs or symptoms that were associated with specific subtypes. The purpose of all of these classification criteria was to provide acceptable homogeneity of groups of children for study of the pathogenesis and aetiology of these diseases, their responses to treatment, and expected outcomes. The ability to anticipate the course and outcome of subgroups of these children would not only benefit a child with the disease in consideration of appropriate treatment regimens, but also be valuable to socio-economic agencies in planning approaches to the health care of children with chronic illnesses.

However, the intrinsic strengths and weaknesses of classification criteria are often overlooked.[26,27] As stated, they serve to identify children with reasonably similar types of arthritis for study, and to separate these children from those who have other clinically defined types of arthritis and courses of disease. In this regard, a distinction needs to be made between *classification criteria* and *diagnostic criteria*. These would be identical if the selection of children with a specific type of disease resulted in criteria that were 100% sensitive and 100% specific. However, it is obvious to any experienced clinician that all of our present criteria either exclude a proportion of patients with that disease at onset, or include a number identified later in their course who have been misclassified.

It was clear in the computer-derived criteria of the 1986 ACR classification[11] that each of the subsets of children identified had different probabilities of correct subclassification. Most important, these data were derived from a clinic population in which diseases classified under the term JRA were frequent (approximately 50% of long-term patients). However, if these same criteria are applied to the population at large, in which these disorders are infrequent (an approximate incidence of 9.2 to 19.6 per 100 000 children),[1,23,28–31] their positive predictive value becomes far less certain. Therein arises a distinct problem for paediatric rheumatology, and that is identifying children with these forms of arthritis in epidemiological surveys, in order to determine the socioeconomic impact of these diseases in a health-care system – a very inefficient task!

It should be emphasized that these difficulties are not pertinent simply to criteria for the childhood age group, but also represent confounding factors in the diagnosis of adult illnesses such as rheumatoid arthritis (RA). For instance, a study by Mitchell and Fries in 1982[32] identified seven major clinical syndromes that were included as RA by the ACR criteria first published in 1958[33] and later modified, and the fact that the relationship between seropositive and seronegative disease remained ambiguous. It was also evident in the Tecumseh Community Health Study that the majority of adults with RA were not characterized by rheumatoid factor seropositivity (70 of 380 persons, 18%),[34] in contrast to patients with RA presenting to a university rheumatology clinic (approximately 85% seropositive).

With all of these factors considered, it becomes difficult and laborious from longitudinal data sets to arrive at classification criteria that are reliable, have face, content, and convergent validity, and are able to identify changes in the course of disease over time that may be clues to differing pathogenic factors or aetiologies.

PURPOSES OF PRECISE NOMENCLATURE

As previously stated, the purpose of a specific name for a disease is to enhance communication among various groups that are concerned with that disorder, including the patient, parents, physicians, local and national support groups, and health-care agencies; and ensure reasonable homogeneity of patients for scientific investigations of aetiology and pathogenesis, and treatment responses to drugs, such as those carried out by the Pediatric Rheumatology Collaborative Study Clinics.[35] It is self-evident that there would be distinct advantages to a uniform international nomenclature instead of the current use of the overlapping terms JRA, JCA, and JA that has become increasingly unclear, imprecise, and confusing in our literature. Unfortunately, the process of choosing names has not only involved incomplete scientific understanding, but has also been confounded by language, culture, pre-existing usage, and national institutions. Perhaps our abortive attempts to consider all of these factors in the choice of a single term has been at the root of the international problem. Furthermore, although it has been difficult to rationalize a designation for use universally in the Western languages, what do we do about the multiplicity of world languages? It has already been mentioned that medical usage in North America, beginning in approximately 1946, has rather consistently used the term JRA for the group of children with idiopathic peripheral arthritis.[8] At this time, that is the term included in the major textbooks of paediatrics in the USA and those of both adult and paediatric rheumatology.[5] A similar usage of JCA is pervasive in some of the European countries, particularly the UK and France.[2,13,14,28,36] Furthermore, a term such as JA was preempted in the USA as a designation for all of the rheumatic diseases of children by the National Foundation in the 1960s in their support of Special Treatment Centers for Juvenile Arthritis. It was later adopted by the Arthritis Foundation in 1980 as the name for the American Juvenile Arthritis Organization, an umbrella association for parents of children with the various rheumatic diseases of childhood and health professionals concerned with their care.

Perhaps in our deliberations we should give more consideration to these cultural factors over which the medical community has little control, or will not have pervasive influence, until precise aetiologies can be identified, as was the case with the discovery of Lyme arthritis as one of the causes of peripheral arthritis in children, a disease very similar in onset to JRA and initially misidentified as such in the New England states.[37] A central question thereby arises of whether we should even try to achieve a universal designation of these diseases, or be willing to conclude that each nation and culture should continue to use their accepted terms. It would be my conclusion that such is the case, and that to attempt to rename these diseases by fiat in the absence of scientific imperatives would be disruptive in the least, not universally accepted, and counterproductive to the nascent interests of paediatric rheumatology as the smallest of the paediatric subspecialties recognized by the American Board of Pediatrics.

Table 12.5 Tentative ILAR classification of idiopathic arthritides of childhood

Polyarthritis, RF-negative
Polyarthritis, RF-positive
Oligoarthritis
Extended oligoarthritis
Systemic arthritis
Psoriatic arthritis
Enthesitis-associated arthritis

RF, rheumatoid factor.
From reference 21.

PURPOSES OF STUDIES OF CLASSIFICATIONS

We should, nevertheless, be able to re-examine the classification of these diseases, particularly the extended course subtypes, in continuing efforts to increase the sensitivity and specificity of existing criteria. It is that task that the ILAR subcommittee has set out to accomplish.[21] In Table 12.5 are listed the seven subtypes of idiopathic arthritis of children that were selected by the ILAR Committee for study. A comparison of Table 12.5 with Table 12.2 indicates that systemic onset was to be evaluated without consideration as to the course subtypes of oligoarthritis or polyarthritis; that oligoarthritis be examined in terms of antinuclear antibody seropositivity and an extended oligoarthritis that included polyarthritis but not necessarily rheumatoid factor seropositivity; and that polyarthritis be considered in terms of rheumatoid factor seropositivity or seronegativity. The committee also recommended that two types of arthritis excluded from the ACR classification be included: enthesitis-related arthritis and psoriatic arthritis. Reasons for not examining all of the course subtypes identified in the 1986 ACR criteria study were not provided,[12] although the committee did not intend that their study would encompass all of the types of idiopathic arthritis in children. Within the ILAR proposal were recommended a number of exclusions, abbreviated definitions, and the admonition that a careful and formalized process of evaluation and annual review be proposed for these tentative criteria, and that they should not be used in publications until they were validated and accepted by the constituent organizations. A number of commentaries have already been published concerning this proposal.[38,39]

An initial effort at evaluation took place this year at the Paris Conference on HLA Typing.

Table 12.6 Population surveys (1994) of children with juvenile rheumatoid arthritis

	Bowyer (n = 1619)	Denardo et al. (n = 914)
Oligoarticular arthritis (JOA) (714.32)	826 (51%)	486 (53%)
Polyarticular arthritis (JPA) (714.33)	536 (33%)	268 (29%)
RF-negative	—	239 (26%)
RF-positive	—	29 (3%)
Systemic onset arthritis (JSA) (714.31)	257 (16%)	146 (16%)
Definite	—	111 (12%)
Probable	—	35 (4%)
Unclassified arthritis	—	14 (2%)

From references 41 and 42.

Much attention has been focused on the relationship of the HLA genes of the major histocompatibility complex with the types of arthritis that develop in children, and presumably in part to their pathogenesis.[40] However, it is clear that HLA typing is limited in its utility as a clinical tool for classification in that the precise roles of the HLA genes in pathogenesis are unknown. These genes are incompletely penetrant, specific identified mutations appear to be few, and an enormous degree of polymorphism exists. Their validity as criteria is most limited by the ethnic and genetic background of the population studied. However, the naming of these genes, although complex and constantly changing, has not been controversial; the scientific community can be certain that a specific gene when studied will be the same around the world, irrespective of the ethnic group under consideration. In fact, the nomenclature of the HLA genes is a good illustration of the lack of controversy in an area of medical science when its developments are exclusively confined to the scientific arena, and have not been contaminated by the difficulties of language or lay usurpation.

The limited utility of HLA typing can be illustrated by an examination of the frequency of the onset types of JRA in population surveys. In Table 12.6 are listed data on the three onset types based upon population surveys of children with JRA conducted in the USA in 26 paediatric rheumatology clinics by Bowyer for 1992–1994, (S Bowyer, personal communication), and by Denardo et al for an 8-year period in paediatric rheumatology clinics in Southern New England.[41] The remarkable similarity of the frequency of these onset types in these two studies is striking (and similar to data from the ACR 1986 study): juvenile oligoarticular arthritis, 51% and 53%, juvenile polyarticular arthritis, 33% and 29%, and juvenile systemic arthritis, 16% in both series. However, similar data from Canada and Europe need to be compared in order to construct a sense of the comparability, or lack of comparability, of the various populations that might be studied by HLA typing. For instance, an investigation from Manitoba, Canada, by Oen and associates[42] of Aboriginal children with arthritis provided a strikingly different frequency for rheumatoid-factor-seropositive polyarticular disease (29 of 61, 48%) from that identified in Caucasian children in the same clinic, and a different sense of the occurrence of HLA-DR4 or DR8 subtypes, e.g. there was no statistical association of rheumatoid-factor-positive and polyarticular JRA with DRB1*0404 because of the high frequency of this specificity in controls (22% vs 36%). These data underscore the profound diversity that is going to be found in differing ethnic groups.

CLINICAL USAGE

How might current names of these disorders be used in our clinics with patients and their families? The term *arthritis* seems to be the one in North America that is associated with a connotation of fear for the child or family. A paediatric rheumatologist needs, therefore, to spend a considerable amount of time and an adequate period of counselling to provide as much encouraging information to the family as can honestly be cited. This process depends upon accurate subsetting of disease, and careful, but not overextended, prognostication for selection of treatment regimens. *Rheumatoid* is a designation that most of our parents would have difficulty defining. The term *chronic*, although accurate scientifically, is one that most North American families have difficulty accepting at onset. I have found that it is best left out of our discussion for at least the first few clinic visits. *Juvenile* seems to be well understood, particularly when the family has joined the American Juvenile Arthritis Organization, or the local AJAO chapter of the Arthritis Foundation, and certainly after they have attended one of the annual or regional meetings of this organization.

I assume that all paediatric rheumatologists subset their patients for parents or referring physicians into the children with polyarthritis, those with oligoarthritis, or those with systemic disease. It becomes easy then to avoid using either 'rheumatoid' or 'chronic' if we simply characterize a child as having polyarticular arthritis, oligoarticular arthritis, or systemic arthritis, perhaps with the prefix 'juvenile' in order to emphasize the differences between these diseases and adult RA. Abbreviations such as JPA, JOA, and JSA continue the tradition in both medicine and bureaucracies, of finding abbreviations for virtually any frequently used designation.

CONCLUSIONS

A reasonable conclusion might be that first, we lay to rest for the moment any recommendations for a change of the terms that have evolved in various countries and cultures for idiopathic peripheral arthritis of children. Second, we should continue to define precisely the classification criteria used in publications on children with arthritis. In other words, JRA is a term that can only be understood in terms of the ACR classification criteria[11] (and has a different meaning in the EULAR criteria), and JCA is a term that must be referenced to the EULAR criteria.[13] JA has no defining criteria and will continue to be used by the lay public and organizations in varying ways within specific geographic regions. Third, as recommended by the ILAR committee,[22] their proposed designations and criteria should not be used in publications except those directed at defining and validating their subsets. For example, criteria for specific disorders that have been validated, e.g. the Vancouver criteria for psoriatic arthritis,[17] should continue to be used, until they are shown to be less sensitive or specific than newly developed definitions of the ILAR committee.

A consensus that appears to be unchallenged has emerged from all of the controversy surrounding the nomenclature of idiopathic peripheral arthritis in children during the past 25 years. This consensus is that (1) an international agreement on nomenclature not only is highly desirable but eventually will be required, (2) classification criteria and nomenclature defining the varying subgroups of arthritis in children must be tested prospectively and validated, and (3) any change in nomenclature must be adopted on a strictly scientific basis. It is time that we separate considerations of language, culture, and continental imperatives from this controversy. To quote William James: 'There can be no final truth in ethics anymore than in physics until the last man has had his experience and said his say.'[43]

REFERENCES

1. Cassidy JT, Petty RE. *Textbook of Pediatric Rheumatology*. WB Saunders: Philadelphia, 1995.
2. Prieur A-M. What's in a name? Nomenclature of juvenile arthritis. A European view. *J Rheumatol* 1993; **20** (Suppl 40):10–11.
3. Southwood TR, Woo P. Childhood arthritis: the name game. *Br J Rheumatol* 1993; **32**:421.
4. Laxer RM. What's in a name: the nomenclature of juvenile arthritis. *J Rheumatol* 1993; **20** (Suppl 40):2–3.
5. Cassidy JT. What's in a name? Nomenclature of juvenile arthritis. A North American view. *J Rheumatol* 1993; **20** (Suppl 40):1–5.
6. Hanson V. From Still's disease and JRA to JCPA, JCA, and JA: medical progress or biased ascertainment? *J Rheumatol* 1982; **9**(6):819–20.
7. Prieur A-M, Petty RE. Definitions and classifications of chronic arthritis in children. *Baillière's Clin Paediatr* 1993; **1**:695.
8. Coss JA Jr, Boots RH. Juvenile rheumatoid arthritis. A study of fifty-six cases with a note on skeletal changes. *J Pediatr* 1946; **29**:143–56.
9. Brewer EJ Jr, Bass JC, Cassidy JT et al. Criteria for the classification of juvenile rheumatoid arthritis. *Bull Rheum Dis* 1972; **23**:712–19.
10. Brewer EJ Jr, Bass J, Baum J et al. Current proposed revision of JRA criteria. *Arthritis Rheum* 1977; **12** (Suppl 10):195–9.
11. Cassidy JT, Levinson JE, Bass JC et al. A study of classification citeria for a diagnosis of juvenile rheumatoid arthritis. *Arthritis Rheum* 1986; **29**:274–81.
12. Cassidy JT, Levinson JE, Brewer EJ Jr. The development of classification criteria for children with juvenile rheumatoid arthritis. *Bull Rheum Dis* 1989; **38**:1–7.
13. Wood PHN. Special meeting on nomenclature and classification of arthritis in children. In: *The Care of Rheumatic Children* (Munthe E, ed.). EULAR Publications: Basel, 1978:47–50.
14. Prieur AM, Ansell BM, Bardfeld R et al. Is onset type evaluated during the first 3 months of disease satisfactory for defining the sub-groups of juvenile chronic arthritis? A EULAR Cooperative Study (1983–1986). *Clin Exp Rheumatol* 1990; **8**:321–5.
15. Prieur A-M, Listrat V, Dougados M et al. Evaluation of the ESSG and the Amor criteria for juvenile spondylarthropathies (JSA). Study of 310 consecutive children referred to one pediatric rheumatology center [abstract]. *Arthritis Rheum* 1990; **35**:D159.
16. Petty RE. Juvenile psoriatic arthritis, or juvenile arthritis with psoriasis? *Clin Exp Rheumatol* 1994; **12** (Suppl 10):S55–S58.
17. Ansell BM, Bywaters EGL. Prognosis in Still's disease. *Bull Rheum Dis* 1959; **9**:189–92.
18. Ansell BM, Bywaters EGL. Diagnosis of 'probable' Still's disease and its outcome. *Ann Rheum Dis* 1962; **21**:253–62.
19. Bywaters EGL. Diagnostic criteria for Still's disease (juvenile RA). In: *Population Studies of the Rheumatic Diseases, Proceedings of the Third International Symposium* (Bennett PH, Wood PHN, eds.). Excerpta Medica: Amsterdam, 1968: 235–40.
20. Ansell BM, Wood PHN. Prognosis in juvenile chronic polyarthritis. *Clin Rheumat Dis* 1976; **2**:397–407.
21. Fink CW. The Task Force for Classification Criteria: proposal for the development of classification criteria for idiopathic arthritides of childhood. *J Rheumatol* 1995; **22**:1566–9.
22. Kvien TK, Hoyeraal HM, Kass E. Diagnostic criteria of rheumatoid arthritis in children: proposed criteria for controlled clinical studies. *Scand J Rheumatol* 1982; **11**:187–92.
23. Andersson Gäre B, Fasth A, Andersson J et al. Incidence and prevalence of juvenile chronic arthritis: a population survey. *Ann Rheum Dis* 1987; **46**:277–81.
24. Kunnamo I, Kallio P, Pelkonen P. Incidence of arthritis in urban Finnish children. A prospective study. *Arthritis Rheum* 1986; **29**:1232–1238.
25. Cassidy JT, Sullivan DB, Petty RE. Clinical patterns of chronic iridocyclitis in children with

juvenile rheumatoid arthritis. *Arthritis Rheum* 1977; **20**:224–7.

26. Bloch DA, Moses LE, Michel BA. Statistical approaches to classification: methods for developing classification and other criteria rules. *Arthritis Rheum* 1990; **33**:1137–44.
27. Fries JF, Hochberg MC, Medsger TA Jr et al. Criteria for rheumatic disease: different types and different functions. *Arthritis Rheum* 1994; **27**:454–62.
28. Andersson Gäre B. Juvenile chronic arthritis. A population based study on epidemiology, natural history and outcome. Department of Pediatrics, University of Göteborg, Sweden, 1994.
29. Sullivan DB, Cassidy JT, Petty RE. Pathogenic implications of age of onset in juvenile rheumatoid arthritis. *Arthritis Rheum* 1975; **18**:251–5.
30. Towner SR, Michet CJ Jr, O'Fallon WM, Nelson AM. The epidemiology of juvenile rheumatoid arthritis in Rochester, Minnesota 1960–1979. *Arthritis Rheum* 1983; **26**:1208–13.
31. Peterson LS, Mason T, Nelson AM, O'Fallon WM, Gabriel SE. Juvenile rheumatoid arthritis in Rochester, Minnesota 1960–1993. Is the epidemiology changing? *Arthritis Rheum* 1996; **39**:1385–90.
32. Mitchell DM, Fries JF. An analysis of the American Rheumatism Association criteria for rheumatoid arthritis. *Arthritis Rheum* 1982; **25**:481–7.
33. Ropes MW, Bennett GA, Cobb S et al. 1958 revision of diagnostic criteria for rheumatoid arthritis. *Bull Rheum Dis* 1958; **9**:175–6.
34. Mikkleson WM, Dodge HJ, Duff IF, Epstein FH, Napier JA. Clinical and serological estimates of the prevalence of rheumatoid arthritis in the population of Tecumseh, Michigan, 1959–60. In: *The Epidemiology of Chronic Rheumatism* (Kellgren J, ed.). IFA Davis: Philadelphia, 1963: 239–48.
35. Brewer EJ Jr, Giannini EH, Standard methodology for segment I, II, and III Pediatric Rheumatology Collaborative Study Group studies. I. Design. *J Rheumatol* 1982; **9**:109–13.
36. Dequeker J, Mardjuadi A. Prognostic factors in juvenile chronic arthritis. *J Rheumatol* 1982; **9**:909–15.
37. Athreya BH, Rose CD. Lyme disease. *Curr Prob Pediatr* 1996; **26**:189–207.
38. Hochberg MC. Classification criteria for childhood arthritic diseases [editorial]. *J Rheumatol* 1995; **22**:1445–6.
39. Malleson P. Proposal for classification criteria for idiopathic arthritides of childhood [letter]. *J Rheumatol* 1996; **23**:942.
40. De Inocencio J, Giannini EH, Glass DN. Can genetic markers contribute to the classification of juvenile rheumatoid arthritis? *J Rheumatol* 1993; **20** (Suppl 40):12–18.
41. Denardo BA, Tucker LB, Miller LC et al. Demography of a regional pediatric rheumatology patient population. *J Rheumatol* 1994; **21**:1553–61.
42. Oen K, Schroeder ML, Jacobson K, Anderson S. Immunogenetics of JRA in a Canadian aboriginal population [abstract]. *Arthritis Rheum* 1996; **39** (Suppl 9):53.
43. James W. *Essays in Pragmatism* (edited with an introduction by A Castell). Hafner: New York, 1948.

13

Does infection cause chronic arthritis in children?

Taunton R Southwood

INTRODUCTION

The search for the aetiology of chronic inflammatory joint disease in children is one of the great challenges in rheumatology. In a landmark review, Wallace and Levinson demonstrated that the long-term outcome of such disease was poor, and significant lifelong physical disability was the end result in over 30% of cases.[1] In fact, with a prevalence rate of 1 in 1000 children, chronic arthritis is one of the commonest causes of physical disability in childhood. It is likely that therapeutic control, or even prevention, of this disease will be possible only if we can arrive at a greater understanding of the aetiology and pathogenesis of chronic childhood arthritis.

Research efforts in this area have been hampered in the past by inconsistencies and incongruities in disease classification, particularly between the umbrella definitions of juvenile chronic arthritis (JCA) used in Europe and juvenile rheumatoid arthritis (JRA) used in North America (reviewed in reference 2). This is discussed in more detail in Chapter 12. A further potential source of confusion is the rather arbitrary nature of the distinction between adult and childhood forms of chronic arthritis. There is a large body of data concerning the role of infection in the aetiology of adult rheumatoid arthritis and spondylarthritis which will not be discussed in this chapter, even though some of it may be relevant to the understanding of childhood arthritis.

For the purposes of the current chapter, the term JCA will be used for the chronic idiopathic arthritides of childhood, and the subgroups of *pauciarticular onset* [those (1) beginning before (early onset) or (2) after (late onset) 6 years of age; (3) associated with psoriasis; or (4) progressing to polyarthritis], *polyarticular onset*, and *systemic onset* JCA will be considered where appropriate. It must be emphasized that significant associations with aetiologic (possibly infectious) agents may be obscured unless research programmes analyse data which are well matched to biologically homogeneous disease groups.

The aim of this chapter is to explore the possibility that JCA is caused by infectious agents. The first section will briefly review the laboratory techniques that have been used to search for an infectious aetiology in JCA, and the second section will discuss the histopathology of the synovium in JCA from an infection-related viewpoint. The following sections will deal with the subgroups of JCA in relation to the infectious agents with which each has been associated. The concluding section will examine the possible pathogenic mechanisms for chronic arthritis in relation to an infectious aetiology.

TECHNIQUES THAT HAVE BEEN USED TO IMPLICATE INFECTION IN JCA

Microbial culture

The distinctions between septic arthritis, reactive arthritis, and most forms of chronic arthritis in children are important in understanding the spectrum of the association between arthritis and infection. By definition, JCA is idiopathic.[3] The demonstration of an infectious aetiology for any arthritis should result in the designation of that disease to distinguish it from JCA. Septic arthritis, characterized by the recovery of viable infectious agents (typically bacteria) from the synovial space, undoubtedly occurs in children and its sequelae of cartilaginous and bony destruction may result in longstanding joint disease.[4,5] However, this diagnosis is relatively rare, and accounts for less than 5% of children with rheumatic disease in the UK.[6] Reactive arthritis is probably much more common. It is defined as an arthritis in which the joint fluid is sterile, but evidence of a concurrent or immediately preceding infection is demonstrated in extra-articular tissues or fluid.

In the vast majority of children with chronic arthritis, viable infectious agents cannot be recovered from the synovial space and therefore joint sepsis in the conventional sense is very unlikely. There are, however, examples of potential overlap between JCA, reactive arthritis and septic arthritis. One famous example is Lyme arthritis, in which a group of children originally thought to have JCA were found to have infection with *Borrelia burgdorferi*.[7] Spirochetes can be isolated from synovial tissue, but it is unlikely that this organism plays a major role in JCA; *B. burgdorferi* DNA could not be detected by means of the polymerase chain reaction (PCR) in synovial fluid samples from 20 patients with JCA, and immune responses to the antigens could not be demonstrated in a large series of JCA patients.[8–11] Brucellar arthritis may also be difficult to distinguish from JCA.[12] It is unclear whether either of these diseases represents true septic arthritis or reactive arthritic processes, but both may have chronic clinical manifestations. Even more confusing is the relationship between JCA and viral infection. Viable rubella virus has been recovered from the synovial fluid and peripheral blood mononuclear cells of a small number of children with JCA.[13] Does this, therefore, represent septic arthritis?

Techniques for demonstrating intra-articular antigens

In adult patients with reactive arthritis, many microbial antigens have been detected in synovial tissue by means of PCR, in situ hybridization or immunofluorescent techniques; these include *Chlamydia trachomatis, Salmonella enteriditis, Salmonella typhimurium, Shigella flexneri, Yersinia enterocolitica* and *Yersinia pseudotuberculosis*.[14] Similar studies in children have not been reported, perhaps because it is rare that synovial tissue from children is available for such techniques. Synovial fluid cells are more readily accessible and may reflect the cellular composition of synovial tissue, but again there have been few studies looking for specific intra-articular antigens. It is probable that advances in technology will yield positive findings; for example, evidence of *C. trachomatis* DNA has been found in a small number of JCA patients, with the use of nested PCR techniques (G Kingsley, personal communication).[15] It is also possible that the isolation of 'new' organisms may provide further insight into chronic inflammatory illnesses such as JCA, as has been suggested for the recently recognized association between hepatitis C virus and autoimmune disease.[16]

Immunity against infectious agents

To demonstrate a causal relationship between infection and JCA in the absence of the ability to fulfil Koch's postulates by microbial culture and reculture, one would need to demonstrate that:

- exposure to an agent preceded the onset of the disease and there was a high relative risk of developing the disease after exposure;
- laboratory evidence of infection was a consistent finding in different patients and different laboratories; and
- specific treatment of the agent resulted in a reduction of disease activity.

Children are exposed to a wide range of wild type and attenuated infectious agents, and virtually every event in childhood is preceded by an infection of some sort! In a case–control study, Kunnamo used a parent-completed questionnaire to record evidence of an upper respiratory infection occurring within 1 month of the onset of JCA.[17] Just over 60% of patients had such symptoms, compared to a third of normal controls and 50% of children with orthopaedic problems. Given this frequency of exposure, one of the strongest arguments against a causal link between infection and JCA is the relative rarity of arthritis during childhood. In other words, the vast majority of childhood infections and immunizations must carry a very low relative risk for arthritic complications.[18,19] Similarly, additional protection against infection, for example in breast-fed infants, has not been shown to prevent the occurrence of JCA.[20] Epidemiological studies may lead to further insights into such relationships. In the paediatric population of Manitoba, Canada, fluctuations in mycoplasma infection over a period of several years were found to correlate closely with variations in the incidence of JCA.[21]

An indirect laboratory method of assessing exposure to an infectious agent is to quantify the immune responses to that agent, either by measuring specific antibodies or mononuclear cell proliferation on re-exposure to the agent in the laboratory. Demonstration of an increased precursor frequency of synovial T cells recognizing that antigen (with the use of limiting dilution techniques) would provide further evidence implicating the antigen in the aetiology of the disease. There is anecdotal evidence that proliferation of synovial fluid mononuclear cells appears to reflect the inciting arthritogenic agent in juvenile reactive arthritis.[22] However, such responses may alter, depending on the length of time between the onset of arthritis and the sampling of the synovial fluid.[23] T cell proliferative responses in isolation may not provide reliable evidence of a putative aetiological infectious agent in children with chronic arthritis.

THE HISTOPATHOLOGY OF THE SYNOVIUM IN JCA

The principal histological finding in JCA is hyperplasia of the synovium.[24] This, together with hyperaemia and subsynovial oedema, accounts for the hypertrophic appearance of the synovium, which eventually forms frond-like villi, extending into the joint space. The key question which needs to be addressed in the context of this chapter is: can an infectious aetiology provide a biologically plausible explanation for the synovial pathology?

Many groups have demonstrated that, in JCA, irrespective of the subtype, the predominant immune cell infiltrating the synovium is the activated CD4+ T cell, expressing transferrin receptors, interleukin (IL)-2 receptors, VLA-1 antigens and MHC class II antigens.[25–28] T cells expressing the gamma delta TCR (approximately 10% of T cells in the JCA joint) also express activation antigens.[29] The primary function of the T cells is to coordinate an immune response to exogenous antigens; in other words, it is entirely possible that the influx of activated T cells into the JCA joint is a process driven by an exogenous, foreign antigen.[30]

The T-cell surface molecule that imparts antigen specificity is the T-cell receptor. If the immune response in the joint was antigen driven, one would expect an intra-articular expansion of a relatively small number of T-cell families (synovial oligoclonality) when compared with the T-cell receptor repertoire in peripheral blood.[31] At least three groups have found evidence supporting this hypothesis;[32–34] in particular, Doherty et al[33] found that the T-cell receptor families Vβ2, Vβ6, Vβ8, and Vβ20 appeared to be overexposed in the synovial fluid in five patients with JCA (four were HLA-B27 positive). Thompson et al assessed synovial fluid samples in 36 patients with JCA (13 with early onset pauciarticular disease, five with late onset pauciarthritis, 14 with polyarthritis and four with systemic disease) and found that the polyarticular patients expressed a higher number of diverse clones, whereas pauciarticular disease was associated with Vβ20 clonal expansion.[34] It is unclear whether samples taken at different stages in the disease process express different patterns of clonality.

Further (albeit indirect) support for an antigen-driven pathogenesis in JCA comes from the observation that the synovial CD4+ T cells in JCA tend to be grouped in contact with dendritic cells, the most important antigen-presenting cells.[35] These cells are likely to express on their cell surface the antigens from any relevant infectious agents responsible for initiating or perpetuating JCA. This and the preceding observations suggest that an infectious aetiology can provide a plausible explanation for the synovial pathology.

However, there are arguments against the hypothesis of an intra-articular antigen-driven T-cell influx. Firstly, it is possible that the accumulation of a limited number of families of activated T cells in the joint may be the result of an antigen nonspecific process. Synovial inflammation is associated with the upregulation of cell adhesion molecules on high endothelial venules, the main portal for T cells to enter the joint. This process would favour the accumulation of activated memory T cells in the synovium, independent of any particular inciting antigen, which would nevertheless result in an altered intrasynovial T-cell repertoire compared to that in peripheral blood. Silverman et al demonstrated that there are increased numbers of the CD45RO-positive T-cell subset (memory phenotype), expressing CD29 (a migration or homing receptor) in the joint.[28] It is possible that the driving force for the accumulation of these cells was the inflammatory process itself, independent of antigen initiation.

The second argument against an infectious aetiology is that no research group has been able to demonstrate convincingly the presence of intra-articular foreign antigens in JCA synovium. There is no doubt that the synovium is an important component of the reticuloendothelial system, and it is clear that the joint is vulnerable to invasion by foreign antigens.[36] It is also probable that the presence of these antigens in the joint is dependent on the length of time which elapses between disease onset and synovial tissue sampling. A project specifically aimed at obtaining synovial tissue from children with JCA within the first few weeks of arthritis onset may have a greater chance of revealing intra-articular antigens.

CLINICAL SUBGROUPS OF JCA AND THEIR ASSOCIATION WITH INFECTIOUS AGENTS

Pauciarticular onset JCA

This disease affects four joints or fewer during the first 6 months after onset. Although there are at least four important subgroups of this onset type, there have been few reports that differentiate between them in association with infectious agents.

Early-onset disease (beginning before the age of 6 years) is associated with chronic anterior uveitis and the presence of antinuclear antibodies (ANA), and carries a good articular prognosis. In an uncontrolled case series, six children with undifferentiated pauciarticular onset arthritis and eye disease (four patients with subacute arthritis and two with conjunctivitis) were reported to have evidence of *Chlamydia* infection by urethral culture.[37] One of the children had typical chlamydial particles in the synovial fluid, and three children were ANA-positive.

This form of arthritis is associated with several HLA antigens, with the combination of the three alleles DR5, DR8 and DP2.1 conferring a relative risk of 236.5.[38] A fascinating study of the HLA antigens associated with early-onset pauciarticular JCA, DRB1*11 (DR5 split) and DRB1*08 (DR8), demonstrated that this association may be due to the differential ability of these specific alleles to present pathogenic peptides from infectious agents to the immune system.[39] The anchor residues of peptides which bound to the two alleles but not to a third (DRB1*0401, which is negatively associated with this form of arthritis) were determined. Peptides from candidate disease-associated antigens were synthesized, including those from streptococcus, parvovirus B19 and rubella.

They were found to bind directly to DRB1*11 and DRB1*08, suggesting that a structural approach may provide a further avenue to explore the mechanism whereby infection could lead to JCA.

Late-onset pauciarticular arthritis (beginning after 8 years) has a male predominance and usually involves the large joints of the lower limb. This group is likely to represent a juvenile form of spondylarthropathy.[40–42] It is associated with HLA-B27 and also has strong links with infection. Individuals who carry HLA-B27 are up to 100 times more likely to develop arthritis after genitourinary or gastrointestinal infection.[36]

Enteric bacterial infections have been clinically implicated in the aetiology of juvenile reactive arthritis and juvenile spondylarthropathy. Infections with salmonella, shigella, campylobacter or yersinia during childhood may be accompanied by peripheral arthritis, and occasionally by typical Reiter's syndrome (arthritis, urethritis and conjunctivitis). There are anecdotal reports of progression from juvenile reactive arthritis to clinical spondylarthropathy.[23]

Subacute bowel inflammation (histological evidence of acute or chronic ileocolonic inflammation) is found in up to 80% of patients with juvenile spondylarthropathy or late-onset pauciarticular juvenile chronic arthritis.[43,44] There is also evidence that immune responses to enteric bacteria are found in the synovial compartment of children with juvenile spondylarthropathy. Approximately 90% of children who have HLA-B27-positive chronic arthritis have synovial fluid lymphocyte responses to enteric bacteria, compared with only 25% of children with HLA-B27-negative disease.[45] In addition, up to a fifth of children with overt inflammatory bowel disease develop arthritis. Successful treatment of the bowel inflammation with sulphasalazine may be accompanied by remission of peripheral arthritis; this benefit appears to depend on the antibiotic (sulpha) component, which may alter enteric bacterial colonization.

There are at least two other subgroups of childhood arthritis which begin with pauciarticular disease. Juvenile psoriatic arthritis is often difficult to recognize initially, as the psoriatic rash may not become clinically evident for many years after the onset of arthritis.[46] There have been anecdotal reports of varicella (chicken pox) infection triggering juvenile psoriatic arthritis.[47] There is no other evidence to link infection to this subtype of arthritis at present, although it is intriguing to postulate that commensal skin organisms might be involved. Patients with juvenile psoriatic arthritis may develop arthritis in many joints during the course of the disease, in a pattern similar to that of extended pauciarticular JCA. There are no reports specifically linking this latter group to infection.

Polyarticular-onset JCA

This disease affects more than four joints, usually in a symmetrical fashion, during the first 6 months after onset. There is a female preponderance, and it carries a poorer prognosis than pauciarticular-onset JCA. Early-onset disease (onset before the age of 6 years) is rheumatoid-factor-negative and is associated with HLA-DP3.[48] Late-onset disease (usually in adolescent women before their 16th birthday) is usually rheumatoid-factor-positive and is very similar in clinical features and immunogenetic associations to adult-type rheumatoid arthritis.[49] Polyarticular-onset JCA has been associated with several infectious agents, of which streptococcus, rubella, influenza A and parvovirus will be discussed in more detail.

It is well recognized that streptococcal infection is associated with arthritis in children. One of the criteria for the diagnosis of rheumatic fever is a flitting large joint polyarthritis. However, there have been several reports of isolated poststreptococcal reactive arthritis in children who do not have other features of rheumatic fever.[50,51] It is controversial whether this condition is a separate disease or part of a clinical spectrum with rheumatic fever, as a number of patients with JCA have abnormally high antibody titres to streptococcal antigens.

One of the most fascinating associations between infection and JCA was reported by Chantler et al.[13] She and her colleagues isolated rubella virus from peripheral blood and/or synovial fluid mononuclear cells in seven of 19 JCA patients. Both of the patients with polyarticular-onset JCA carried the virus, compared to one of five patients with systemic JCA, two of six with pauciarticular onset JCA and 2 of 6 with spondylarthritis. Rubella could not be isolated from any normal disease controls, and very few adults with rheumatoid arthritis. The pathogenic significance of this study has been thrown into some doubt recently by the observation that synovial lymphocyte proliferation to rubella virus was rarely observed in children with JCA of any subgroup.[52] A further report investigating the possible occurrence of persistent rubella virus infection did not support the role of rubella virus in this disease.[53] Evidence of the virus was not demonstrated in any of 11 children with JCA, by either culture or PCR. The subgroup of JCA was not specified. In the control group, however, rubella virus was isolated from blood or nasopharyngeal secretions of four subjects following rubella immunization or wild type infection. The PCR detected the virus in three control subjects. The report did not investigate synovial fluid mononuclear cells, which were the cells most often carrying the virus in Chantler's study.

Influenza A is an epidemic virus which undergoes frequent mutations. A particular strain (H2N2) was responsible for an epidemic in the UK during 1963, and Pritchard and Munro reported a group of girls who were born in that year who not only had detectable antibodies to the H2N2 strain, but also had developed chronic erosive polyarthritis.[54] In a double-blind placebo-controlled study, the patients who received the anti-influenza therapy amantidine appeared to improve, although no effect was noted on the levels of virus-specific antibodies. In addition, patients with JCA have been reported to have increased peripheral blood mononuclear cell proliferative responses to influenza A when compared to age-matched controls.[45] All 12 of the patients had more vigorous responses in the synovial cell population than in peripheral blood, raising the possibility that specific immunity to the virus was localized to the joint.

The facial rash of erythema infectiosum is the most common paediatric manifestation of human parvovirus B19 (HPV) infection, a virus which is associated with transient articular manifestations in 80% of adults and 8% of children.[55] This virus has been implicated in the aetiology of rheumatoid arthritis in adults and a recent case report demonstrated both IgM and IgG antibodies to HPV-B19 in a 5-year-old boy with transient knee arthritis, in association with the typical 'slapped cheek' clinical sign of HPV infection.[56,57] A survey of 104 children with acute arthritis in Boston, USA, revealed IgM anti-HPV-B19 antibodies in 20, of whom six went on to develop chronic symptoms indistinguishable from JCA.[58]

Systemic-onset JCA

This is an illness which has no particular sex predilection and may begin at any age (even adulthood!). The predominant clinical features at onset are extra-articular, with daily spiking fever, an erythematous, evanescent rash, hepatomegaly, splenomegaly, lymphadenopathy and occasionally pericarditis or other form of serositis. The accompanying arthritis is often polyarticular in course and may be extremely difficult to control, adding an extra impetus to elucidate the underlying aetiology. Of all the subgroups of JCA, this appears to be most similar clinically to the typical picture of an infectious disease. Particularly suggestive features include the fever, generalized ill health and accompanying laboratory findings of a marked leukocytosis with neutrophilia and left shift towards immature white cells. Unfortunately, convincing scientific evidence implicating infectious agents in systemic-onset JCA is lacking.

There have been several case reports of coxsackievirus associated with this disease in both children and adults. Rising titres to coxsackie A9, B2, B3, and B4 were noted in association with high spiking fever, macular erythematous rash, pericarditis, and chronic arthritis.[59,60] There was a close correlation between the height of the titres to A9 and B3, and exacerbations of the disease in a 16-year-old boy. In the adults, rising titre antibodies to coxsackie B4 have been reported.[61]

Epstein–Barr virus (EBV) has also been implicated in systemic-onset JCA. Twenty-seven of 52 patients with the disease (52%) were found to have antibodies to the viral capsid antigen of EBV, compared to 30% of patients with other forms of JCA and 43% of the control population. The percentage of systemic JCA patients carrying this marker of past EBV infection was even higher in the 5–10-year-old age group (64%), but unfortunately there were no comparable figures for age-matched controls.[62] More recently Tsai et al, using molecular techniques, were unable to demonstrate an increased frequency of EBV or cytomegalovirus in leukocytes from 21 patients with undifferentiated JCA, compared to 20 patients with childhood systemic lupus erythematosus (SLE) and 20 controls.[63]

POSSIBLE PATHOGENIC MECHANISMS FOR THE DEVELOPMENT OF CHRONIC ARTHRITIS IN CHILDREN AFTER AN INFECTION

There are two hypotheses concerning pathogenic mechanisms for the development of chronic arthritis following an infection; these will be explored in this section, on the basis of both experimental evidence and speculation. The first is the possibility that there is a direct link between enteric infection and arthritis, and the second is the possibility that molecular mimicry and cross-reactive immune responses are responsible for the pathogenesis of the disease.

The link between enteric infection and arthritis

It is in the juvenile spondylarthropathies that some of the strongest evidence implicating enteric infectious agents has been demonstrated. These arthritides are linked to the B*2705 subtype of HLA-B27, and advances in molecular techniques have enabled the study of animal models into which this human gene has been introduced. Transgenic Lewis rats expressing a high cell-surface density of human B*2705 develop a peripheral arthritis and spondylarthropathy during the first 6 weeks of life. These features appear to be specific for the B27 gene, as they are not seen in the rats expressing the B*2705 gene in low copy number, or in rats transgenic for HLA-B7.[64] However, the B*2705 gene in isolation is not enough for the development of arthritis; enteric bacteria are also needed to trigger the disease. When maintained in a sterile environment from birth, transgenic rats did not develop either peripheral arthritis or spondylarthropathy.[65] Additionally, the histological evidence of bowel inflammation seen in association with the spondylarthropathy was absent in rats raised under germ-free conditions. Unfortunately, the responsible enteric pathogen or pathogens have yet to be isolated with the use of this model.

It is also possible that the gastrointestinal inflammation may be the result of a defective immune response, as observed in cytokine and T-cell receptor mutant mice.[66] Other hypotheses for the association of the B27 gene with arthritis include presentation of an arthritogenic peptide (which may arise from the B27 gene itself), linkage disequilibrium with more closely disease-associated genes, and reduced immune resistance to enteric bacteria at the level of the antigen-presenting cell.[67–69]

The evidence for a link between the gut and the joint in children with spondylarthropathy stems from the observations made by Mielants et al.[43] They found histological evidence of acute or chronic ileocolonic inflammation in the majority of patients with juvenile spondylarthropathy or the precursor illness of late-onset pauciarticular juvenile chronic arthritis, raising the possibility that an increase in gut wall permeability to enteric pathogens might play a role in the pathogenesis of the arthritis. Children may carry up to 1 kg of bacteria in the gut, and it would be somewhat surprising if an inflamed, presumably compromised, gut mucosal barrier did not predispose to inflammation elsewhere in the body, such as the joints![70] An increase in permeability to [^{51}Cr]EDTA, independent of the use of nonsteroidal anti-inflammatory drugs, has been demonstrated in spondylarthropathy.[71,72]

The question remains: is there a mechanism for migration of inflammatory cells or enteric antigens to the synovium from a presumed site of pathology in the gut mucosa? For example, is intermittent or chronic bacteraemia or antigenaemia responsible for seeding the joint space with pathogenic antigens? An intriguing report has provided evidence for specific lymphocyte migration between gastrointestinal mucosal endothelium and synovial endothelium. Lymphocytes in migration around the body normally gain entry to sites of inflammation via specialized postcapillary blood vessels known as high endothelial venules (HEV). Salmi et al isolated activated mucosal lymphocytes from gut lamina propria and found the cells to bind to the HEV of synovium almost as efficiently as to mucosal HEV, whereas they did not bind to the HEV of peripheral lymph nodes.[73] The molecular nature of the adherence molecules was determined (involving the integrins β7 and α4/β1), and the authors concluded that the dual binding capacity of mucosal lymphocytes may help to explain the pathogenesis of arthritis associated with enteric bacteria. If this were the case, the immune responses to enteric bacteria observed in the synovial lymphocytes from children with spondylarthropathy may not result from direct invasion of the joint by foreign antigens from enteric bacteria.

Molecular mimicry and cross reactive immune responses

Another mechanism to explain the chronicity of childhood arthritis following an acute infection is antigenic similarity (i.e., molecular mimicry) between human proteins and foreign antigens. Were this to be the case, an adaptive immune response generated as a result of an acute infection could conceivably recognize (i.e., cross react with) self-antigens in the synovial cavity and perpetuate a localized chronic inflammatory disease. Candidate foreign antigens have included EBNA-1 from EBV with similarity to a peptide of 107 amino acid residues from collagen and keratin, *Klebsiella pneumoniae* pullulanase, which has an epitope similar to one of collagen, and antigens from various bacteria (klebsiella, yersinia and shigella) which have similarities to HLA-B27 itself.[74–76] These reports have discussed mainly adult arthritis, and will not be discussed further here.

Heat-shock proteins (hsp) have been investigated as potentially cross reactive antigens in JCA. Heat-shock proteins are highly conserved throughout evolution, from bacteria to humans, and appear to act as immunodominant epitopes in many acute infections. In other words, immune responses initially directed against bacterial hsp could cross react with human hsp. The initial work in this field stemmed from the adjuvant arthritis rat model. A clone of T cells recognizing the 180–188 nonapeptide of mycobacterial hsp65 was isolated from an arthritic rat. This clone could transfer the disease to naïve rats, and was found to cross react with a core protein of cartilage proteoglycan.[77] Danieli and colleagues demonstrated that half of JCA patients had peripheral blood lymphocyte responses to the 180–188 nonapeptide of mycobacteral hsp65, but they were not able to demonstrate a close sequence homology between this epitope and the proteoglycan link protein in collagen.[78]

Other bacterial hsp have been implicated in JCA, including the *Escherichia coli* hsp60 (GroEl) and the dnaJ class of hsp.[45,79,80] The latter antigen has been found to contain the QKRAA sequence, which is identical to the 'arthritis motif' in the DRB1 chain of HLA-DR, providing a potential mechanism for cross reactivity. Immune responses to two peptides from dnaJ were documented in peripheral blood and synovial fluid mononuclear cells from adults with rheumatoid arthritis, but not in 18 children with JCA.[79] The GroEl antigen has been shown to induce proliferative responses in children with HLA-B27-positive spondylarthropathies and to a lesser extent in other forms of childhood arthritis. The responses to this antigen correlate very closely to responses to other enteric bacteria including yersinia and salmonella.[55]

There is close sequence homology between enteric bacterial hsp60 and human hsp60, but it is still not known whether T-cell clones recognizing GroEl cross react with the human antigen (Bhayani H, unpublished observations). Immune responses to human hsp65 and expression of hsp65 and hsp70 on synovial membrane have been demonstrated in six patients with JCA, and none of the normal or adult RA controls.[81,82] The majority of immune responses to hsp60 occurred in the early-onset pauciarticular JCA subgroup, particularly during relative disease remission.[83,84] This supports the possibility that immune responses to hsp are part of T-cell regulatory mechanisms controlling the development of arthritis. However, it is unclear whether such hsp are specific to JCA, as they have also been demonstrated in other paediatric inflammatory conditions such as SLE and dermatomyositis.[85] In addition, a fundamental difficulty in the interpretation of data concerning molecular mimicry is understanding how the normal mechanisms of immune tolerance to self-antigens (and therefore to foreign epitopes with sequence homology to self-antigens) are broken down in chronic inflammation and autoimmune disease. The potential role of molecular mimicry in the pathogenesis of spondylarthropathy has been disputed from many quarters.[86] A more detailed analysis of the links between hsps and arthritis is provided in chapter 2.

CONCLUSION

In conclusion, there is compelling evidence, but as yet no proof, that infectious agents are responsible for triggering and perhaps perpetuating the arthritic process in the juvenile spondylarthropathies, particularly in the presence of the genetic background indicated by HLA-B27. In other forms of chronic arthritis in childhood there is controversy and dissent about all aspects of their aetiology, pathogenesis, and even nomenclature. It would be foolhardy indeed to argue too forcefully in support of a role for infection in this diverse group of conditions at present. For the future, I hope to live long enough to understand the answers!

REFERENCES

1. Wallace CA, Levinson JE. Juvenile rheumatoid arthritis: outcome and treatment for the 1990s. *Rheum Dis Clin North Am* 1990; **17**:891–905.
2. Southwood TR, Woo P. Childhood arthritis: the name game. *Br J Rheumatol* 1993; **32**:421–3.
3. Wood PHN. Nomenclature and classification of arthritis in children. In: *The Care of Rheumatic Children* (Munthe E, ed.). EULAR Mongraph. Series 3. EULAR Publications: Basel, 1978:47–50.
4. Paterson DC. Acute suppurative arthritis in infancy and childhood. *J Bone Joint Surg* 1970; **52B**:474–82.
5. Fink CW, Nelson JD. Septic arthritis and osteomyelitis in children. *Clin Rheum Dis* 1986; **12**:423.
6. Symmons D, Jones MA, Osborne J et al. Paediatric rheumatology in the United Kingdom: epidemiological data from the British Paediatric Rheumatology Group National Diagnostic Index. *J Rheumatol* 1996; **23**:1975–80.
7. Szer IS, Taylor E, Steere AC. The long-term course of Lyme arthritis in children. *N Engl J Med* 1991; **325**:159–63.
8. Johnston YE, Duray PH, Steere AC et al. Lyme arthritis: spirochetes found in synovial microangiopathic lesions. *Am J Pathol* 1985; **118**:26–34.
9. Schmidli J, Hunziker T, Moesli P, Schaad UB. Cultivation of *Borrelia burgdorgeri* from joint fluid three months after treatment of facial palsy due to Lyme borreliosis. *J Infect Dis* 1988; **158**:905–6.
10. Malawista SE, Schoen RT, Moore TL et al. Failure of multitarget detection of *Borrelia burgdorferi*-associated DNA sequences in synovial fluids of patients with juvenile rheumatoid arthritis: A cautionary note. *Arthritis Rheum* 1992; **35**:246–7.
11. Banerjee S, Banergee M, Cimolai N et al, Seroprevalence survey of borreliosis in children with chronic arthritis in British Columbia, Canada. *J Rheumatol* 1992; **19**:1620–4.

12. Alvarez De Buergo M, Gomez Reino FJ, Gomez Reino JJ. A long term study of 22 children with brucellar arthritis. *Clin Exp Rheumatol* 1990; **8**:609–12.
13. Chantler JK, Tingle AJ, Petty RE. Persistent rubella virus infection associated with chronic arthritis in children. *N Engl J Med* 1985; **313**:1117–23.
14. Viitanen AM, Arstial RP, Lahesmaa R et al. Application of the polymerase chain reaction and immunofluorescence techniques to the detection of bacteria in yersinia-triggered reactive arthritis. *Arthritis Rheum* 1991; **34**:89–96.
15. Bas S, Griffais R, Kvien TE et al. Amplification of plasmid and chromosome chlamydia DNA in synovial fluid of patients with reactive arthritis and undifferentiated seronegative oligoarthropathies. *Arthritis Rheum* 1995; **38**:1005–13.
16. Pivetti S, Novarino A, Merico F et al. High prevalence of autoimmune phenomena in hepatitis C virus antibody positive patients with lymphoproliferative and connective tissue disorders. *Br J Haematol* 1996; **95** 204–21.
17. Kunnamo I. Infections and related risk factors of arthritis in children: a case control study. *Scand J Rheumatol* 1987; **16**:93–9.
18. Thompson GR, Weiss JJ, Eloise MI et al. Intermittent arthritis following rubella vaccination: A three-year follow-up. *Am J Dis Child* 1973; **125**:526–30.
19. Benjamin CM, Chew GC, Silman AJ. Joint and limb symptoms in children after immunization with measles, mumps and rubella vaccine. *Br Med J* 1992; **304**:1075–8.
20. Rosenberg AM. Evaluation of associations between breast feeding and subsequent development of juvenile rheumatoid arthritis. *J Rheumatol* 1996; **23**:1080–2.
21. Oen K, Fast M, Postle B. Epidemiology of juvenile rheumatoid arthritis in the province of Manitoba. *Arthritis Rheum* 1993; **36** (Suppl 9):61.
22. Southwood TR, Hancock EJ, Petty RE et al, Tuberculosis rheumatism (Poncet's disease) in a child. *Arthritis Rheum* 1988; **31**:1311–13.
23. Southwood TR, Gaston JSH. Evolution of synovial fluid mononuclear cell responses in a HLA B27-positive patient with yersinia-associated juvenile arthritis. *Br J Rheumatol* 1993; **32**:845–8.
24. Bywaters EGL. Pathologic aspects of juvenile chronic polyarthritis. *Arthritis Rheum* 1977; **20**:271–6.
25. Poulter LW, Al-Shakarchi HAA, Campbell EDR et al. Immunocytology of synovial fluid cells may be of diagnostic and prognostic value in arthritis. *Ann Rheum Dis* 1986; **45**:584–90.
26. Odum N, Norling N, Platz P et al. Increased prevalence of late stage T-cell activation antigen (VLA-1) in active juvenile chronic arthritis. *Ann Rheum Dis* 1987; **46**:846–52.
27. Bergroth V, Konttinen YT, Pelkonen P et al. Synovial fluid lymphocytes in different subtypes of juvenile rheumatoid arthritis. *Arthritis Rheum* 1988; **31**:780–3.
28. Silvermann ED, Isacovics B, Petsche D, Laxer RM. Synovial fluid cells in juvenile arthritis: evidence of selective T-cell investigation to inflamed tissues. *Clin Exp Immunol* 1993; **91**:90–5.
29. Kjeldsen-Krach J, Quayle AJ, Vinje O et al. A high proportion of the Vd1+ synovial fluid cd T cells in juvenile rheumatoid arthritis patients express the very early activation marker CD69, but carry the high molecular weight isoform of the leucocyte common antigen (CD45RA). *Clin Exp Immunol* 1993; **91**:202–6.
30. Germain RN. The ins and outs of antigen processing. *Nature* 1986; **322**:687–9.
31. de Maria AF, Malnati MS, Poggi A et al. Clonal analysis of joint fluid T lymphocytes in patients with juvenile rheumatoid arthritis. *J Rheumatol* 1990; **17**:1073–8.
32. Maksymowych HP, Gabriel CA, Luyrink L et al. Polymorphysim in a T-cell receptor variable gene is associated with susceptibility to a juvenile rheumatoid arthritis subset. *Immunogenetics* 1992; **35**:257–62.
33. Doherty PJ, Silverman ED, Laxer RM et al. T-cell receptor Vb usage in synovial fluid of children with arthritis. *J Rheumatol* 1992; **19**:463–8.
34. Thompson SD, Grom AA, Bailey S et al. Patterns of T lymphocyte clonal expansion in HLA-typed patients with juvenile rheumatoid arthritis. *J Rheumatol* 1995; **22**:1356–64.
35. Knight SC. Dendritic cells in inflammatory joint disease. In: *Immunopathogenetic mechanisms of arthritis* (Goodacre J, Carson Dick E eds.). MTP Press, 1989; 69–85.
36. Brewerton DA. Causes of arthritis. *Lancet* 1988; **2**:1063–6.
37. Maximov A, Shaikow AV, Lovell DJ et al. Chlamydial associated syndrome of arthritis and eye involvement in young children. *J Rheumatol* 1992; **19**:1794–7.

38. Paul C, Schoenwald U, Truckenbrodt H et al. HLA-DP/DR interaction in early onset pauciarticular juvenile chronic arthritis. *Immunogenetics* 1992; **37**:442–8.
39. Nepom B. Structural characteristics of peptides binding preferentially to pauciarticular onset JRA-associated HLA alleles. *Arthritis Rheum* 1995; **38** (Suppl 9):308.
40. Rosenberg AM, Petty RE. A syndrome of seronegative enthesopathy and arthropathy in children. *Arthritis Rheum* 1982; **25**:1041–7.
41. Cabral DA, Oen KG, Petty RE. SEA syndrome revisited: a longterm follow-up of children with a syndrome of seronegative enthesopathy and arthropathy. *J Rheumatol* 1992; **19**:1282–5.
42. Burgos-Vagas R, Clark P. Axial involvement in the seronegative enthesopathy and arthropathy syndrome and its progression to ankylosing spondylitis. *J Rheumatol* 1989; **16**:192–7.
43. Mielants H, Veys EM, Joos R et al. Late onset pauciarticular juvenile chronic arthritis relation to gut inflammation. *J Rheumatol* 1987; **14**:459–65.
44. Mielants H, Veys EM, Goemaere S et al. A prospective study of patients with spondyloarthropathy with special reference to HLA B27 and to gut histology. *J Rheumatol* 1993; **20**:1353–8.
45. Life PF, Hassell A, Williams K et al. Responses to gram negative enteric bacterial antigens by synovial T cells from patients with juvenile chronic arthritis: recognition of heat shock protein HSP60. *J Rheumatol* 1993; **20**:1388–96.
46. Southwood TR, Petty RE, Malleson PN et al. Psoriatic arthritis in children. *Arthritis Rheum* 1989:**32**:1007–13.
47. Shore A, Ansell BM. Juvenile psoriatic arthritis – an analysis of 60 cases. *J Pediatr* 1982; **74**:505–16.
48. Fernandez-Vina MA, Fink CW, Sang S, Stastny P. Peptide transporter genes in susceptibility to persistent pauciarticular juvenile arthritis. *Arthritis Rheum* 1993; **36**: (Suppl S54):95.
49. Nepom BS. The role of the major histocompatibility complex in autoimmunity. *Clin Immunol Immunopathol* 1993; **67**:S50–S55.
50. Goldsmith DP, Long SS. Post streptococcal disease of childhood – a changing syndrome. *Arthritis Rheum* 1982; **25** (suppl 14):S18.
51. Fink CW. The role of the streptococcus in poststreptococcal reactive arthrtis and childhood polyarteritis nodosa. *J Rheumatol* 1991; **18** (Suppl 29):14–20.
52. Pugh MT, Southwood TR, Gaston JSH. Paediatric rheumatology: review. The role of infection in juvenile chronic arthritis. *Br J Rheumatol* 1993; **32**:838–44.
53. Frenkel LM, Nielsen K, Garakian A et al. A search for persistent rubella virus infection in persons with chronic symptoms after rubella and rubella immunization and in patients with juvenile rheumatoid arthritis. *Clin Infect Dis* 1996; **22**:287–94.
54. Pritchard MH, Munro J. Successful treatment of juvenile chronic arthritis with a specific antiviral agent. *Br J Rheumatol* 1989; **28**:521–7.
55. Ager EA, Chin TDY, Poland JD. Epidemic erythema infectiousum. *N Engl J Med* 1966; **275**:1326–31.
56. White G, Mortimer PP, Blake DR. Human parvovirus arthropathy. *Lancet* 1985; **i**:419–21.
57. Rivier G, Gerster C, Terrier P Cheseaux JJ. Parvovirus B19 associated monoarthritis in a 5 year old boy. *J Rheumatol* 1995; **22**:766–7.
58. Nocton JJ, Miller LC, Tucker LB, Schaller JG. Human parvovirus B19-associated arthritis in children. *J Pediatr* 1993; **122**(2):186–90.
59. Rahal JJ, Millian SJ, Noriega ER. Coxsackievirus and adenovirus infection: Association with acute febrile and juvenile rheumatoloid arthritis. *J Am Med Assoc* 1976; **235**:2496–501.
60. Heaton DC, Moller PW. Still's disease associated with Coxsackie infection and haemophagocytic syndrome. *Ann Rheum Dis* 1985; **4**:341–4.
61. Roberts-Thomson PJ, Southwood TR, Smith MD et al. Adult-onset Stills disease or Coxsackie polyarthritis. *Aust NZ J Med* 1986; **16**:509–11.
62. Gear AJ, Venables PJW, Edwards JMB et al. Rheumatoid arthritis, juvenile arthritis, iridocyclitis and the Epstein–Barr virus. *Ann Rheum Dis* 1986; **45**:6–8.
63. Tsai YT, Chiang BL, Kao YF et al. Detection of Epstein–Barr virus and cytomegalovirus genome in white blood cells from patients with juvenile rheumatoid arthritis and childhood systemic lupus erythematosus. *Int Arch Allergy Immunol* 1995; **106**:235–340.
64. Hammer RE, Maika SD, Richardson JA et al. Spontaneous inflammatory disease in transgenic rats expressing HLA-B27 and human β_2m: An animal model if HLA-B27-associated human disorders. *Cell* 1991; **63**:1099–112.
65. Taurog JD, Richardson JA, Croft JT et al. The germfree state prevents development of gut and joint inflammatory disease in HLA-B27 transgenic rats. *J Exp Med* 1994; **180**:2359–64.

66. Strober W, Ehrhardt RO. Chronic intestinal inflammation: and unexpected outcome in cytokine or T-cell receptor mutant mice. *Cell* 1993; **75**:203–5.
67. Hermann E, Fleischer B, Meyer zum Buschenfelde KH. Bacteria-specific cytotoxic CD8+ T cells: a missing link in the pathogenesis of the HLA-B27-associated spondylarthropathies. *Ann Med* 1994; **26**:365–9.
68. Benjamin R, Parham P. HLA-B27 and disease: a consequence of inadvertent antigen presentation? *Rheum Dis Clin North Am* 1992; **18**:11–20.
69. Khare SD, Harvinder SL, David CS. Spontaneous inflammatory arthritis in HLA-B27 transgenic mice lacking β_2-microglobulin: a model of human spondyloarthropathies. *J Exp Med* 1995; **182**:1153–8.
70. Lahesmaa-Rantala R, Magnusson KE, Granfors K et al. Intestinal permeability in patients with yersinia triggered reactive arthritis. *Ann Rheum Dis* 1991; **50**:91–4.
71. Mielants H, Goemaere S, De Vos M et al. Intestinal mucosal permeability in inflammatory rheumatic diseases. I. Role of antiinflammatory drugs. *J Rheumatol* 1990; **18**:389–93.
72. Mielants H, de Vos M, Goemaere S et al. Intestinal mucosal permeability in inflammatory rheumatic diseases. II. Role of disease. *J Rheumatol* 1990; **18**:394–400.
73. Salmi M, Andrew DP, Butcher EC, Jalkanen S. Dual binding capacity of musosal immunoblasts to mucosal and synovial endothelium in humans: dissection of the molecular mechanisms. *J Exp Med* 1995; **181**:137–49.
74. Sulitzeanu D, Anafi M. EBV, molecular mimicry and rheumatoid arthritis: a hypothesis. *Immunol Lett* 1989; **20**:89–92.
75. Fielder M, Pirt SJ, Tarpey I et al. Molecular mimicry and ankylosing spondylitis: possible role of a novel sequence in pullulanase of *Klebsiella pneumoniae. FEBS Lett* 1995; **369**:243–8.
76. Gaston JSH. How does HLA-B27 confer susceptibility to inflammatory arthritis? *Clin Exp Immunol* 1990; **82**:1–2.
77. van Eden W, Holoshitz J, Nevo Z et al. Arthritis induced by a T-lymphocyte clone that responds to *Mycobacterium tuberulosis* and to cartilage proteoglycans. *Proc Natl Acad Sci* 1985; **82**:5117–20.
78. Danieli MG, Markovits D, Gabrielli A et al. Juvenile rheumatoid arthritis patients manifest immune reactivity to the mycobacterial 65 kDa heat shock protein, to its 180–199 peptide and to a partially homologous peptide of the proteoglycan link protein. *Clin Immunol Immunopathol* 1992; **64**:121–8.
79. Albani S, Andree G, La Cava A et al. The Epstein–Barr virus (EBV) mimics the three HLA alleles mainly related to early onset pauciarticular juvenile rheumatoid arthritis (JRA). *Arthritis Rheum*1993; **36** (suppl 9):207.
80. Albani S, Keystone EC, Nelson JL et al. Positive selection in autoimmunity: Abnormal immune responses to a bacterial dnaJ antigenic determinant in patients with early rheumatoid arthritis. *Nature Med* 1995; **1**:448–52.
81. de Graeff-Meeder ER, Van Der Zee R, Rijkers GT et al. Recognition of human 60 kD heat shock protein by mononuclear cells from patients with juvenile chronic arthritis. *Lancet* 1991; **337**:1368–72.
82. Boog CJP, De Graeff-Meeder ER, Lucassen MA et al. Two monoclonal antibodies generated against human hsp60 show reactivity with synovial membranes of patients with juvenile chronic arthritis. *J Exp Med* 1992; **175**:1805–10.
83. Prakken ABJ, Rijes GT, Toebes EA et al. Reactivity to hsp60 in the onset of oligoarticular JCA. *Arthritis Rheum* 1993; **36** (Suppl 9):207.
84. de Graeff-Meeder ER, van Eden W, Rijkers GT et al. Juvenile chronic arthritis: T-cell reactivity to human hsp60 in patients with a favourable course of arthritis. *J Clin Invest* 1995; **95**:934–40.
85. Conroy SE, Tucker L, Latchman DS, Isenberg DA. Incidence of anti-hsp90 and 70 antibodies in children with SLE, juvenile dermatomyositis and juvenile chronic arthritis. *Clin Exp Rheum* 1996; **14**:99–104.
86. Lahesmaa R, Skurnik M, Granfors K et al. Molecular mimicry in the pathogenesis of spondyloarthropathies. A critical appraisal of cross-reactivity between microbial antigens and HLA-B27. *Br J Rheumatol* 1992; **31**:221–9.

14

Why are children with juvenile rheumatoid arthritis small?

Philip J Hashkes and Daniel J Lovell

One of the unique outcomes of chronic childhood diseases is the retardation of physical growth. Growth failure, described by some as 'dwarfism',[1,2] is one of the less frequently mentioned and more disturbing permanent sequelae seen in juvenile rheumatoid arthritis (JRA) or juvenile chronic arthritis (JCA), as labelled in Europe. We have used JRA in this chapter unless JCA was specifically mentioned in a quoted article (see Chapter 12).

The fact that some children with JRA are 'small' was mentioned in 1897 by George Frederic Still, who in his classical description of juvenile arthritis noted 'the general arrest of development that occurs when the disease begins before the second dentition'.[3] Kuhns and Swaim described three types of growth disturbance in JRA: (1) generalized retardation of growth; (2) persistence of infantile proportions and appearance of the extremities; and (3) localized limb growth abnormalities.[1] This chapter will focus on generalized retardation of growth.

Much still remains controversial or unknown in the investigation of why children with JRA are 'small'. The first question to be answered is the truth of that assumption in the 1990s. Many of the original studies were from an era in which effective treatment options were few and corticosteroid use was widespread. Most studies did not follow patients to adulthood and were therefore unable to report fully on the growth outcome in JRA. Data analysis such as the definition of 'small' and measurement of height in patients with joint deformities and asymmetric limb length may also affect results.

The causes of growth failure in JRA are multiple and have not been elucidated completely. These include disease activity, nutritional deficiencies, the effect of medications, specifically corticosteroids, and hormonal deficiencies (mainly growth hormone (GH) and other growth factors).

Furthermore, only preliminary intervention studies have been performed in an effort to increase height and weight in JRA. Only rudimentary reports exist on the effect of increased disease control by use of more aggressive pharmacological agents or the effect of nutritional supplementation. Several studies of GH supplementation have been performed. However, long-term controlled studies are still lacking. Successful interventional trials will undoubtly shed further light on the aetiology of 'smallness' in JRA.

This chapter reviews much of what is known about growth deficiencies in JRA and outlines what is controversial and issues that remain to be investigated.

INTRODUCTION TO JRA

JRA is a group of chronic idiopathic arthritides in children with disease onset at or before the age of 16 years (also see chapter 12). Three distinct onset subtypes have been identified based on the clinical manifestations in the first 6 months of disease. Pauciarticular-onset JRA is the most common, involving four or fewer joints and is seen in 50% of patients. Polyarticular-onset JRA, involving five or more joints, is seen in 40% of patients.

Systemic-onset JRA, seen in 10% of patients, is characterized by daily spiking fevers greater than 103°F (39.4°C) and the appearance of a fleeting erythematous rash. The associated arthritis may develop long after the onset of fever.

JRA is the most common of the paediatric rheumatic diseases, and is the most common cause of arthritis in childhood. The estimated annual incidence of JRA is 0.9 cases per 10 000 children in the USA and the prevalence is approximately 1 per 1000.[4,5] With a population of approximately 65 000 000 children aged less than 16-years in the USA,[6] approximately 65 000 children in the USA have JRA.

HOW PREVALENT ARE GROWTH DISTURBANCES IN JRA?

Many case reports of growth failure followed the description by Still. However, in the early study by Kuhns and Swaim only one of 12 patients was reported to be shorter than the lower limit of age- and sex-matched norms.[1]

Later studies found a much greater prevalence of growth disturbances. The first longitudinal study was by Ansell and Bywaters.[7] The weight of 119 and height of 113 hospital-referred patients with Still's disease were observed over 5 years, between 1948 and 1953. Height was not measured in six patients with hip or knee flexion deformities. The weight of 48% of the patients was more than 10% below the normal mean of age and sex controls. Weight loss occurred early in the disease, and tended to correct itself with remission, mainly in patients with disease duration of less than 3 years. Height was less affected than weight. The minimum height recorded was 80% of the normal mean. In only 12% of patients was height more than 10% below the normal mean. Duration of disease and disease activity were the most important factors, with height returning to normal within 2 to 3 years of remission, if the epiphyses were not fused. Corticosteroid therapy (see discussion below) was associated strongly with lower height.

Bernstein et al were the first to examine serial height data for the separate subtypes of JRA.[8] They followed 31 patients for an average of 6.6 years. The mean changes in height in polyarticular- and pauciarticular-onset were 0.2 and 0.3 percentiles, respectively. However, the mean change in patients with systemic-onset JRA was –6.7 percentiles ($P < 0.01$). Eleven of the 13 patients with systemic-onset JRA had received corticosteroids. Overall, the height of 40% of patients was below the 3rd percentile, significantly more than expected for the age-matched general population ($P < 0.0005$). At disease onset, 33% of the patients were below the 3rd percentile, also significantly more than the age-matched general population ($P < 0.005$).

Other studies found significant growth retardation in patients not treated with corticosteroids who had polyarticular-onset JRA. Bacon et al examined 56 patients randomly chosen from their clinic population.[9] The mean height for age of the systemic-onset and polyarticular-onset groups were the 31.5 and 34.9 percentiles, respectively. Weight for age was decreased significantly only in the polyarticular-onset group (28.6 percentile; $P < 0.01$). Weight for height was decreased in the polyarticular-onset group (32 percentile; $P < 0.01$), but was above normal in the systemic-onset group (69.7 percentile). This study, which was the first to integrate measurement of weight and height, suggested that nutritional factors relating to weight loss may influence height gain as well.

Data on growth were collected in several long-term observational studies. Most series reported on hospitalized patients or patients seen in a tertiary centre. Therefore, patients with more severe disease were more likely to be reported. In a series from Germany of 433 hospitalized children, followed for an average of 15 years between 1952 and 1979, the height of 10% of 209 patients with systemic-onset JCA was below the 3rd percentile.[2] The epiphyseal lines of most patients were closed. Therefore, the height of most patients was representative of their adult outcome. In a series from Sweden, Svantesson et al followed 33 hospitalized patients with systemic-onset JRA for 4–24 years (median 10 years).[10] Thirteen patients had growth retardation (height or weight was

Table 14.1 Disease characteristics of 103 patients with juvenile rheumatoid arthritis

	Systemic		Polyarticular		Pauciarticular	
	n	%	*n*	%	*n*	%
Disease onset	21	20.4	40	38.8	42	40.8
Disease course	5	4.8	62	60.2	36	35.0

unspecified) greater than 3 standard deviations below the normal mean. Twelve developed JRA before the age of 5 and all were treated with daily corticosteroids for more than 4 years.

These studies did not report specifically on the height outcome attained following epiphyseal fusion. Delayed puberty seen in adolescents with JRA is a possible pitfall.[7] In one study, menarche was delayed by nearly 1 year ($P < 0.015$).[11] Johansson et al found short stature only in patients younger than 13 years of age, whereas older patients had heights similar to those of controls.[12] Thus, JRA patients may continue to grow later than the general population.

Lovell and White[13] examined the adult heights of patients from the Cincinnati database of the American Rheumatism Association Medical Information Service (ARAMIS). Height data were obtained from 156 patients followed past the age of 18. Overall, 17% of the patients were below the 5th percentile, and 50% of systemic-onset, 16% of polyarticular-onset and 11% of pauciarticular-onset patients were below the 5th percentile. Although the use of corticosteroids was correlated significantly with growth failure, 58% of the growth failure patients were never treated with corticosteroids.

Questions remain as to whether these findings are correct and applicable to the entire JRA population, not only to hospitalized patients or those referred to a tertiary centre. A recent community-based study from five counties in southwestern Sweden looked at the natural history and outcome of 133 patients with JCA followed until patients reached a median age of 17.7 years.[14] The cohort consisted of patients born between 1968 and 1972 and was studied between 1984 and 1992. Although 49% continued to have active disease requiring medication, no patients were more than 2 standard deviations below the height for the age-comparable general population. As this study was community based, only 3.2% had systemic-onset and 29% polyarticular-onset disease.

As part of the preparation for writing this chapter, we performed a cross-sectional study of 103 consecutive outpatients with JRA seen in the paediatric rheumatology clinic at the University of Cincinnati (PJ Hashkes and DJ Lovell, unpublished data). Sixty-one were female (59.2%) and 42 were male (40.8%). The patients' age, disease duration, onset, and course-type, and past or present use of corticosteroids or methotrexate were recorded. The height on the day of examination was measured by means of a Harpenden stadiometer and weight was measured with a floor-model beam electronic scale. The height and weight percentiles were plotted on age-appropriate growth charts adopted from the National Center for Health Statistics.[15]

Disease characteristics are presented in Table 14.1, and treatment details in Table 14.2. The mean height, weight and percentiles by disease subtype are presented in Table 14.3, and the height and weight percentile distribution by disease subtype are shown in Figures 14.1 and 14.2.

The patients' mean age was 12.3 (standard deviation = 6.2; median = 12.6) years; disease

Table 14.2 Treatment of 103 patients with juvenile rheumatoid arthritis

	Yes		No	
	n	%	*n*	%
Methotrexate at present	49	47.6	54	52.4
Methotrexate in the past	59	57.3	44	42.7
Corticosteroid at present	8	7.8	95	92.2
Corticosteroid in the past	29	28.2	74	71.8

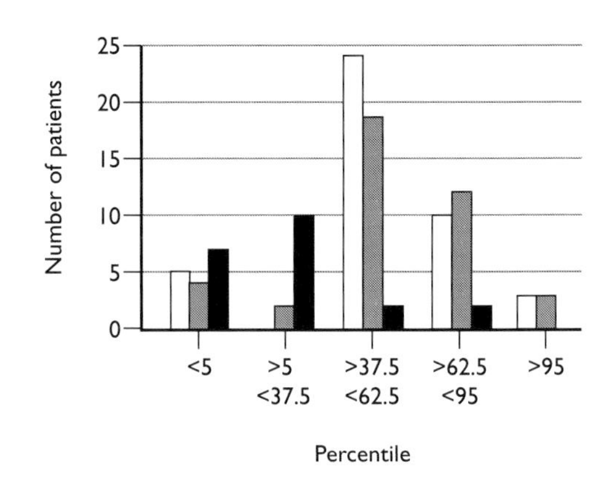

Figure 14.1 Height distribution of 103 patients with juvenile rheumatoid arthritis. □, pauciarticular onset; ▒, polyarticular onset; ■, systemic onset.

duration was 6.8 (5.2; 6.0) years; height was 142.6 (27.7; 148.3) cm; weight was 45.0 (24.9; 39.9) kg; height percentile was 45.7 (31.5; 50) and weight percentile was 53.4 (30.8; 50).

Overall, 16% of the patients were at or below the 5th percentile for height ($P = 0.03$ by chi-square as compared to the normal population) and 8% for weight ($P > 0.3$). When assessed by disease onset, only in systemic-onset JRA were significantly more patients at or below the 5th percentile ($P = 0.006$). The mean height percentile for all patients was 45.7 and for weight it was 53.4. In a comparison of the means among disease subtypes, patients with systemic-onset disease were significantly shorter than those with polyarticular-onset disease, and they were shorter and weighed less than patients with pauciarticular disease (Table 14.3). Height percentiles correlated significantly with disease subtype ($r = 0.299$, $P = 0.002$) and corticosteroid therapy ($r = 0.467$, $P < 0.001$), but not with disease duration ($r = 0.027$, $P > 0.3$). Weight was correlated significantly only with disease subtype ($r = 0.285$, $P = 0.003$), but not with corticosteroid therapy ($r = 0.16$, $P = 0.11$) or disease duration ($r = 0.069$, $P > 0.3$).

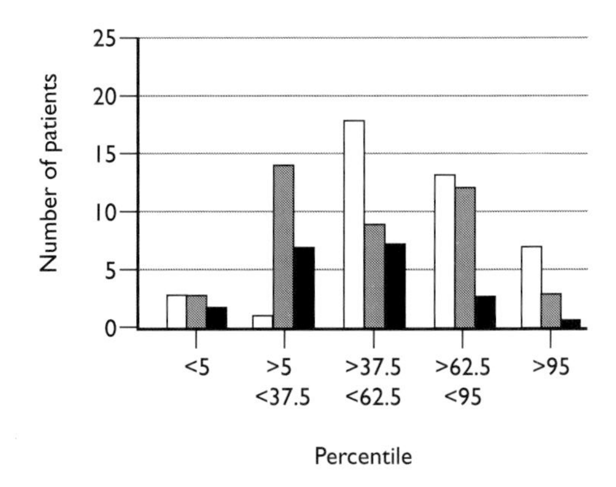

Figure 14.2 Weight distribution of 103 patients with juvenile rheumatoid arthritis. □, pauciarticular onset; ▒, polyarticular onset; ■, systemic onset.

This study confirms previous findings regarding the association of short stature with systemic-onset disease and corticosteroid therapy. However, height was not decreased in other JRA subtypes, and weight was not decreased when compared to the normal

Table 14.3 Comparison of height and weight percentiles between onset subtypes of juvenile rheumatoid arthritis.

Disease onset	*n*	Height percentile		Weight percentile	
		Mean (SD)	Median	Mean (SD)	Median
Systemic	21	21.3 (29.1)	8	40.2 (29.8)	35
Polyarticular	40	53.2 (29.6)	50	50.2 (30.1)	45
Pauciarticular	42	50.8 (29.9)	50	63.0 (29.5)	62.5

Unpaired Student's *t*-test produced the following results for comparisons of systemic vs polyarticular: height percentile, $P < 0.001$; weight percentile, $P = 0.22$; systemic vs pauciarticular: height percentile, $P < 0.001$; weight percentile, $P = 0.005$; polyarticular vs pauciarticular: height percentile, $P > 0.3$; weight percentile, $P = 0.056$.

population in any of the subtypes. Furthermore, the mean height and weight percentile of our cohort was nearly normal, and the number of patients below the 5th percentile was less than in most previous studies.

These last two studies raise doubts about whether it is correct to characterize all children with JRA as 'small' when in reality only a subset of JRA patients are actually 'small', and most patients grow normally.

SPECIFIC ASPECTS OF HEIGHT MEASUREMENT IN JRA

In an excellent article, Cameron[16] has reviewed the complexities of accurate height assessment in normal humans and in various pathologic states. Special problems complicate height measurement in JRA. Patients with hip or knee deformities require special measurement approaches. Inaccuracies of height measurement can also be due to scoliosis from hip deformities or secondary to arthritis of the spinal column. In a study from Sweden, 5.3% of JRA patients had scoliosis greater than 15°, 10 times the rate of the general population.[17] Discrepancies in leg length, commonly seen in pauciarticular-onset JRA, can be significant and result in measurement inaccuracies.[18] Several techniques can be utilized to overcome these problems. Sitting height, measured with a sitting platform, is an excellent alternative for patients with hip or knee contractures. For leg asymmetry, construction of a supporting board to compensate for the shorter leg can help achieve an erect standing position.[16] Alternatively, height can be measured while the subject is only standing on the unaffected leg. It is difficult to correct for scoliosis without the help of radiographs, especially in patients with progressive disease.

The definition of 'small' needs clarification and standardization. For growth hormone (GH) studies, significant growth retardation is defined as more than 3.5 standard deviations below the mean for age, with borderline retardation between –2.5 and –3.5 standard deviations.[19] This definition is appropriate before undertaking an expensive treatment with potential side-effects. However, 'small' may also be thought of in social terms. One does not have to be more than 3.5 standard deviations below the norm to be teased by peers. The definition is not uniform among JRA investigators. Most use height and weight percentiles adopted from local norms. However, the data obtained were reported in multiple ways. Investigators used standard deviations from the mean,[10,14] the average percentile of the group,[9] and the proportion of patients below a certain percentile – the 40th,[7] the 5th,[13] or the 3rd.[2] Others used the raw height or weight measurements. This method was applied more in cross-sectional studies.[12] In longitudinal studies growth velocity was used as a measure of comparison.[8] In studies in which growth is reported as an outcome measure, actual growth should also be compared to expected growth, with the use of parental data rather than a simple report of percentiles.

THE AETIOLOGY OF GROWTH FAILURE

The causes of growth retardation in JRA are multiple and it is usually impossible to identify a single factor as the cause in an individual patient. These factors include the disease process itself, malnutrition, corticosteroid therapy, and deficiencies of growth factors and hormones. Many of these factors are intertwined and influence one another. For example, increased disease activity may result in anorexia secondary to secretion of appetite-depressing cytokines,[20] resulting in nutritional deficits,[9,21] which cause a decrease in the levels of insulin-like growth factors (IGF).[22,23] Patients with severe disease, especially systemic-onset disease, are more often treated with corticosteroids, exacerbating disease-related height loss. Several of the factors associated with growth retardation are well known, but others have only begun to be investigated. For the sake of simplicity each factor will be described separately.

Disease-related factors

It is clear that growth retardation parallels disease activity, becoming worse during flares with the potential of corrective 'catch up' within 2–3 years of remission.[7–9,24] Weight and height loss often develop early in the disease process. For example, 40% of patients followed by Ansell and Bywaters had significant weight loss during the first year of disease.[7] The height of 33% of the patients studied by Bernstein et al was less than the 3rd percentile when they were first seen before therapy was initiated.[8] The risk of height loss is increased further with prolonged disease.[7,8,24] Furthermore, height retardation appears to be associated with disease subtype, the greatest degree of growth retardation being seen in systemic-onset[8,12] and to a lesser degree in polyarticular disease.[9,12,13] Weight loss appears to be more significant in polyarticular disease, due in part to the greater proportion of patients with systemic-onset disease treated with corticosteroids.[9]

Height loss in JRA may be more severe than that seen in other paediatric rheumatic diseases. Bernstein et al found a significantly lower height velocity in patients with JRA compared to patients with systemic lupus erythematosus treated with equivalent disease-suppressive doses of corticosteroids ($P < 0.05$).[8]

Possible disease-related mechanisms include immobilization leading to osteoporosis and retardation of bone formation. Epiphyseal damage and premature closure may result from inflammation. Furthermore, inflammatory mediators may disturb normal patterns of growth.[19]

Long-term outcome studies have not been undertaken to assess whether the use of advanced medications for disease control improves growth. The short-term effect of methotrexate was studied by Hunt et al[25] in 12 prepubertal patients with polyarticular or systemic JRA. Height velocity during the first year of therapy was increased in eight patients and decreased in three patients when compared to the year prior to methotrexate initiation ($P = 0.003$). An increase in the height for age from the 43rd to the 48th percentile was observed ($P = 0.003$).

Nutritional factors

Nutritional status in JRA

Although weight loss in JRA has been noted for many years,[1,7,26,27] only recently have specific studies of the nutritional status in JRA been performed. Weight loss related to malnutrition in JRA may have a more significant impact on body composition than protein–calorie malnutrition in otherwise healthy children. Weight loss in individuals without an associated inflammatory condition involves 90% adipose tissue and 10% lean body mass. In patients with an underlying inflammatory condition, such as JRA, 50% of the weight loss is from lean body mass.[28] Therefore, minor weight loss in JRA may dramatically affect protein stores.

The nutritional status in JCA was first assessed by Johansson et al,[12] who compared a convenience sample of 26 girls with JCA aged 11–16 years with 28 healthy age-matched controls. Anthropometric measurements representing somatic protein stores, such as mid-arm circumference and arm muscle circumference, were decreased in patients with systemic and polyarticular-onset JCA ($P < 0.001$ for all comparisons). However, triceps skinfold thickness, an index of subcutaneous fat stores, was increased. These findings were subsequently confirmed by other investigations, which included random patient samples.[29–32]

Laboratory evidence of malnutrition in JRA is also commonly found. Low levels of albumin,[12] prealbumin,[9,12,29,31,32] and retinol binding protein,[9,32] indicative of depleted visceral proteins, are seen commonly in polyarticular and systemic-onset patients. Prealbumin and retinol binding protein are shorter half-life proteins, and are earlier and more sensitive indicators of protein deficiency than albumin. In the study by Henderson et al,[32] 100% of malnourished patients had prealbumin and retinol binding protein below 2 standard deviations of normal, while albumin was deficient in only 50%. Although active inflammation can also reduce levels of these proteins as part of diversion of the liver activity towards production of acute phase reactants, dietary replenishment results in normalization of visceral protein levels despite ongoing active disease.[13,21] Other vitamin and trace metal serum deficiencies are seen despite adequate intake.[9] These include vitamins A,[9] C,[9] and E,[9] and selenium,[12] zinc[9,21] and iron.[12,21]

Based on various combinations of anthropometric measurements (height, weight, body mass index, plotted percentiles, skinfold thickness, and arm circumference) and biochemical abnormalities (prealbumin, albumin, and retinol binding protein), protein–calorie malnutrition is seen in 19–47% of JRA patients, mainly in systemic or polyarticular-onset disease.[12,29,31] However, Henderson and Lovell found that three of 10 patients with pauciarticular-onset disease had significant nutritional deficits.[31]

The cause of the high prevalence of malnutrition is still not clear. Doubt exists as to whether dietary intake is decreased. Johansson et al did not find differences in dietary intake between JRA and control groups.[12] Similarly, Haugen et al found polyarticular-onset patients to have lower weight than pauciarticular-onset patients and healthy controls, despite increased calorie intake ($P = 0.04$).[21] On the other hand, in a study of 34 JRA patients, Bacon et al found the calorie intake of more than 50% of systemic-onset and 33% of polyarticular-onset patients to be less than the recommended allowance for their age and weight.[9] The diet quality, measured as the ratio of calorie, protein, and other nutrient intake to recommended levels, was below 0.85 in 38% of systemic-onset, 36% of polyarticular-onset and 18% of pauciarticular-onset patients, but not in controls.[9] Similarly, Miller et al reported the mean calorie intake for 18 JRA patients as 50–80% of recommended dietary allowances.[33] Mortensen et al found significantly low calorie intake in patients with systemic ($P < 0.01$) and polyarticular-onset JCA ($P < 0.001$).[34] Several investigators found dietary deficiencies in specific vitamins and trace elements: vitamin E,[9] zinc,[9,21,34] iron,[9,21,33] and calcium.[21,33,34]

Many factors can contribute to anorexia and decreased intake in JRA. Chronic inflammation causes fatigue and poor appetite, perhaps related to increased cytokine production, particularly of interleukin-1 and tumour necrosis factor.[20] Most medications used in JRA, including non-steroidal anti-inflammatory drugs (NSAIDs), methotrexate, hydroxychloroquine, and sulphasalazine, can produce gastrointestinal symptoms in many patients and asymptomatic loss of appetite in young children. Arthritis of the temporomandibular joint, seen in 18–30% of patients, can produce pain with chewing. Malalignment of teeth, which occurs in 20–30% of these patients, can cause further difficulties in chewing and swallowing.[35] Upper extremity arthritis can also make it difficult to prepare meals and use eating utensils.

It has been hypothesized that patients with JRA have increased metabolic needs similar to those of patients following burns or trauma. The association of disease activity and low weight was thought to be related to the increased metabolism from inflammation.[7] Haugen et al found that polyarticular-onset patients weighed less than controls, despite increased dietary intake.[21] However, Lovell et al found that actual energy requirements in JRA patients measured by indirect calorimetry were not statistically different from those estimated by other methods.[29]

Other possibilities such as limited absorption of nutrients from the gastrointestinal tract or altered utilization of nutrients, as seen in other rheumatic diseases, have not been described in JRA. Corticosteroid therapy may contribute to degradation of muscle to provide amino acids for gluconeogenesis. This would cause depletion of somatic protein stores in addition to increased deposition of subcutaneous fat induced by corticosteroids.

The relationship of malnutrition to growth: the effect of prevention and nutritional supplementation

Although the cause and effect relationship of nutritional deficits to weight loss is well established,[9,29,31,34] the effect of nutritional deficiencies on height growth in JRA patients is less clear. Bacon et al did not find a correlation between dietary intake, nutritional status and height.[9] Similarly, Haugen et al did not find short stature in polyarticular-onset patients, although they had significantly lower weights.[21] Although 80% of malnourished patients studied by Henderson and Lovell weighed less than the 5th percentile, only 30% had heights below the 5th percentile.[31] However, in another study, Lovell et al found both height and weight below the 5th percentile in 40% of patients with malnutrition.[29] Mortessen et al found a significant correlation of caloric intake and height.[34] Further evidence that malnutrition affects height was found in preliminary results from the only nutritional intervention study reported in JRA. Lovell and Henderson introduced nocturnal nasogastric feeding to seven patients with moderate to severe protein–calorie malnutrition in whom efforts to increase volitional oral intake failed.[13,36] A 6-month course of nutritional replenishment resulted in an increase of height velocity from 0.15 to 1.62 cm/month and weight velocity from –0.22 to 0.8 kg/month. Somatic and visceral protein stores were normalized in all patients. This programme was well tolerated by the patients and easily administered by parents. This study suggests that aggressive repletion of nutritional deficits may correct height deficits as well as weight. Even if the results of this study are confirmed in larger samples, several questions still remain. How long does nasogastric feeding need to be continued? As long as JRA remains active? The experience in Cincinnati suggests that tube feeding may be required by patients with JRA during periods of active articular disease. Suppression of inflammation either by drugs or by spontaneous improvement is associated with an increased appetite. Will these growth gains continue upon long-term follow-up?

What would be the effect of early detection and treatment of inadequate dietary intake before growth failure? Henderson et al described a simple screening test that was selected to be suitable for routine clinical care.[32] Arm circumference below the 10th percentile for age and sex norms was 80% sensitive and 86% specific in detecting protein–energy malnutrition in patients with JRA. Other measures that can be employed in an attempt to improve oral intake include drugs to treat gastritis and reduce gastrointestinal symptoms related to medication; counselling by trained dieticians to provide nutritional guidelines and suggestions for dietary supplementation;

recommendations by occupational therapists to assist in meal preparation and in providing adaptive eating utensils, and orthodontic care for temporomandibular arthritis.

Factors related to corticosteroid-induced growth delays

Corticosteroids are known to be growth inhibitors. Blodgett et al[37] observed a decrease in height velocity in allergy patients within weeks of treatment with cortisone in doses greater than 45 mg/m^2 per day. Shortly after, Ansell and Bywaters[7] observed a similar phenomenon in JCA. They followed 18 patients treated with doses of cortisone of 25–150 mg/day for at least 3 months. The critical dose that inhibited height gain was 37.5 mg/day in children less than 5 years of age and 50 mg/day in older children. Growth failure and resumption of growth were dependent only on the dose of cortisone, not on disease activity. Laaksonen[24] found that corticosteroid therapy completely 'flattened' the growth curve which was reduced but increasing before therapy was initiated. She reported the threshold of prednisolone to be 6 mg/m^2 per day for more than 6 months. Shorter periods even at somewhat higher doses did not result in growth retardation.

Although the effect of corticosteroids on growth is not specific to JRA, it may be greater in JRA than in other rheumatic diseases. Bernstein et al[8] compared 11 patients treated with corticosteroids to 13 patients similarly treated for systemic lupus erythematosus. The mean rate of growth was significantly more decreased in the 2.8 years of follow-up for the JRA patients (–8.0 percentiles) than for the 2.2 years for lupus patients (–2.5 percentiles) ($P < 0.05$).

The growth-inhibiting effect of corticosteroids depends on several factors, including the pharmacological preparation, dosage scheduling, and individual variations. In a comparative study in asthma by Van Metre et al,[38] cortisone was compared to prednisone. Cortisone was one-fifth as potent in relieving symptoms, but the growth-inhibition effect of cortisone was only one-tenth of that of prednisone. In general, preparations with a longer half-life have greater growth-suppression properties.[39]

The effect of adrenocorticotrophic hormone (ACTH) on growth inhibition is less clear. Zutshi et al found that use of ACTH, rather than oral corticosteroid, as the initial therapy enabled normal growth in six of seven patients.[40] However, less promising results were found both by Zutshi et al and by Sturge et al when ACTH replaced daily prednisone.[40,41]

Deflazacort, an oxazoline derivative of prednisolone, causes less loss of lumbar spine bone mineralization in JCA patients compared to those treated with prednisone.[42] However, the effect on linear growth is less clear. Loftus et al did not find significant differences in height velocity in a 1-year double-blind study that compared prednisone to deflazacort.[42] In renal transplant patients, replacement of methylprednisolone with deflazacort resulted in significant increases in the height velocity over 2 years.[43]

Alternate-day corticosteroids suppresses growth less than daily administration. Ansell and Bywaters found in 28 patients with polyarticular-onset JCA that a somewhat slowed growth rate can be maintained with 6–30 mg/m^2 prednisone administered in the mornings of alternate days.[44] Growth resumption occurred after 6–12 months in 21 other patients converted from a daily to an alternate-day regime. Byron et al found the height velocity of seven children younger than 5 years of age to be equal to that of age-matched controls when treated with alternate-day steroids up to 1 mg/kg.[45] Overall, 11 of 13 children on alternate-day therapy grew normally. Growth resumption of patients converted from daily prednisone preceded recovery of the hypothalamic–pituitary axis. Although disease control may not be as complete, alternate-day corticosteroids may be an alternative for short patients in a crucial period of linear growth.

Several cellular mechanisms of growth suppression due to corticosteroids have been proposed. Corticosteroid-induced osteopenia and decreased osteoblast metabolic activity may reduce the growth of trabecular bones. There is evidence that IGF activity is reduced following prednisone administration, secondary to IGF inhibitors. In alternate-day therapy, IGF activity was normal on the 'off' day.[46] Corticosteroids may also directly inhibit post-translational modifications of procollagen precursors.[39]

Hormonal deficiencies

Thyroid hormone

Many reports of coexisting autoimmune rheumatic diseases, such as antithyroid antibodies, and thyroid disease are found in adults, and in paediatric systemic lupus erythematosus. In JRA, few cases of autoimmune hypothyroidism, including subclinical disease, have been reported.[47,48] However, the prevalence of antithyroid antibodies among patients with JRA may be greater than in the general population. Yarom et al found antithyroid antibodies in 9.2% of 173 patients with all subtypes of JRA compared to 4.7% reported for healthy children.[48,49] Two patients had subclinical hypothyroidism.

When short stature is investigated in JRA, the possibility of associated hypothyroidism as a contributor to growth failure, although uncommon, should be considered.

Growth hormone

Several studies have shown that GH secretion is normal in most JRA patients, even in patients with extreme short stature. Sturge et al found normal GH levels in 20 patients with systemic-onset JRA following insulin hypoglycaemic stimulation.[41] This cohort included patients treated with various regimes of corticosteroids, ranging from no treatment to 8 mg/day of prednisone. The height of most patients on daily corticosteroids was below the 3rd percentile. Similarly, 17 of 20 patients with short stature studied by Butenandt had a GH increase greater than 4 ng/ml following insulin stimulation.[50] Overnight and 24-h secretion levels were also found to be normal in the majority of patients. Chipman et al found normal 24-h GH secretion in 11 of 13 patients with polyarticular JRA not treated with corticosteroids.[51] All patients had normal GH peaks during sleep. In this study the height of only one patient was less than the 3rd percentile. Falcini and Allen et al also found normal GH levels in 42 of 45 patients.[52,53] Allen et al found an increase in the pulse frequency of GH secretion.[53] The significance was unclear. This could be attributed to abnormal sleep patterns or poor nutrition. Six of these patients also had normal responses to clonidine stimulation. More recently, Davies et al demonstrated normal 24-h GH secretion levels and patterns in 14 patients with polyarticular JRA and severe short stature.[54]

A small subset of patients with partially deficient GH secretion may exist. Allen et al reported the GH levels in seven of 10 patients to be in the range of patients with primary GH deficiency.[53] Two of the patients from Chipman's study and three from Falcini's cohort had low levels of GH.[51,52] Three patients from Butenandt's cohort had abnormal GH responses to stimulation tests.[50] In a recent study, Hopp et al found that three of six patients with short stature had abnormally low 24-h GH secretion.[55] Of the three patients with abnormal GH secretion, two underwent a 2-year trial with exogenous GH, with only marginally accelerated growth. Therefore, the clinical significance of partial GH deficiency in JRA is still not well defined.

Overall, there does not appear to be an increase in the prevalence of classic GH deficiency in JRA. However, individual cases may exist. In our recent experience, eight patients with JRA and short stature underwent stimulation tests and two had classic GH deficiency. It is important, therefore, that these patients with short stature continue to be evaluated for GH deficiency, as in usual clinical practice.

Growth hormone therapy

Despite the data on normal GH secretion in most patients with JRA, several case reports and uncontrolled short-term studies have been performed to assess the effect of GH therapy on height in JRA.[50,55–8] Ward et al demonstrated an increase in growth velocity in one of two prepubertal patients with longstanding corticosteroid-treated systemic-onset JRA treated with GH.[57] The unresponsive patient was treated with higher daily doses of prednisone, 5 vs 3 mg/day. Butenandt gave GH to 20 patients with longstanding JCA treated with alternate-day corticosteroids.[50] He found that height velocity increased in the first year in 15 of the 20 patients, from a mean of 1.9 cm/year to 6.2 cm/year. In nine patients height increased by a normal or greater than normal rate for the appropriate bone age. The increased growth rate persisted in 12 patients who continued therapy for a second year. Height velocity decreased to pretreatment rates in six patients after cessation of GH. Height velocity did not correlate with the dose of GH.

Similar results were found by Svantesson in six patients with systemic- or polyarticular-onset JCA treated with recombinant GH, 0.07–0.2 IU/kg per day.[58] Height velocity increased from 2.8 cm/year before treatment to 6.7 cm/year. Five of the patients demonstrated accelerated growth.

Davies et al treated two groups of 10 prepubertal patients with low (12 IU/m^2 per week) and high (24 IU/m^2 per week) doses of recombinant human GH for 1 year.[54] Most patients were treated with alternate-day prednisone or deflazacort. Normal 24-h GH secretion was demonstrated in all patients. Overall, a mean increase in height velocity of 3.1 cm/year was demonstrated ($P < 0.0001$). The height velocity increased from –3.0 to –0.3 standard deviations below the norm ($P < 0.0001$). The increase was greater with the higher dose of GH ($P = 0.02$). Greater responses were seen in polyarticular or pauciarticular disease as compared to systemic-onset JRA ($P = 0.02$) and in patients with lower C-reactive protein levels ($P = 0.003$). Other studies from JRA and other diseases indicate that the efficacy of GH decreases when prednisone is given in a dose greater than 5 mg/day.[57,59]

Most studies found that GH increases growth velocity. The efficacy appears to be dependent on disease activity and corticosteroid dose. Exogenous GH may overcome peripheral resistance to GH by increasing IGF-1 levels or by direct action on the epiphyseal growth plate. The 'normal' levels of GH seen in JRA may not suffice to overcome peripheral resistance to its activity. An analogy may be made to peripheral insulin resistance and primary hypothyroidism, in which levels of insulin or thyroid stimulating hormone (TSH) are increased to compensate for abnormal peripheral responses to usual hormonal secretion.

Despite the promising results, it is still premature to say whether GH therapy is beneficial in increasing eventual adult height. Six of the patients from Butenandt's series were in puberty when GH treatment was started and two others entered puberty shortly after beginning therapy.[50] Furthermore, nine of the responders had decreased disease activity and corticosteroid dosage during the study period. Four of the patients studied by Svantesson entered puberty soon after study commencement and had somewhat diminished disease activity.[58] In these patients, puberty rather than GH may have been responsible for increased height velocity. It has been suggested that GH may work with sex hormones in precipitating the pubertal growth spurt.[60] In that case, early skeletal maturation from GH use may cause premature fusion of epiphyseal growth plates and decreased eventual adult height. Meticulously planned controlled studies with long-term follow-up until closure of epiphyseal growth plates are needed before it can be determined that the response to GH persists beyond the initial effect and actually increases adult height. Investigators need to control for puberty, disease activity, and corticosteroid therapy when planning the trial.

Insulin-like growth factors

The effects of GH are mediated primarily by second messengers IGF, mainly IGF-1, previously described as somatomedin. IGF-1 was thought to be produced mainly in the liver, but it is evident that much of its production is in the vicinity of target tissues in response to GH secretion. These growth factors act via autocrine, paracrine and endocrine effects on chondrocytes at epiphyseal growth plates, increasing cell proliferation and proteoglycan synthesis. Low IGF-1 levels may be due to deficient GH secretion or to defective peripheral GH action.

Following the GH studies previously discussed, it was hypothesized that GH was defective in producing sufficient IGF. Bennett et al found decreased levels of IGF-1 and IGF-2 in 15 children with systemic-onset JRA when compared to 79 age-matched controls.[61] The decrease was more pronounced in patients not treated with prednisone and in patients with elevated erythrocyte sedimentation rate (ESR). However, in longitudinal studies, no correlation between IGF levels and growth rate was found. Similarly, Allen et al found decreased IGF-1 levels in eight of 23 patients with all subtypes of JRA,[53] but no correlation between IGF-1 and the height velocity. In contrast, Aitman et al found a significant positive correlation between IGF-1 levels and height ($P < 0.01$) and to a lesser degree height velocity ($P < 0.05$) in 32 patients with seronegative polyarticular-onset JCA.[62]

Low levels of IGF-1 are found in malnourished humans. IGF-1 levels decrease by 70% following a 10-day fast in normal humans. There is evidence that malnutrition decreases the number of GH receptors or causes post-receptor resistance.[22,23] However, the association in JRA is disputed. Bennett et al did not rule out the contribution of malnutrition to IGF-1 deficiency, the majority of their patients with deficient IGF-1 levels were of normal weight.[61] Aitman et al did not find IGF to correlate with two nutritional indices: body mass index (BMI) and serum albumin level.[62] Bacon and Falcini et al found normal levels of IGF, despite growth retardation and nutritional abnormalities, in many of their patients.[9,52] On the other hand, Allen et al found IGF-1 levels to be more closely correlated with weight than with height, reflecting a possible link to nutritional status.[53]

Allen et al measured GH secretion and IGF-1 levels concomitantly.[53] In seven of eight patients with significantly decreased IGF-1, overnight GH secretion was normal. In six of these patients normal GH secretion was seen in response to clonidine stimulation. Perhaps IGF deficiencies result from abnormal GH bioactivity rather than from deficient GH secretion.

Further understanding of the relationship of disease, nutrition, and GH to IGF will clarify the role IGF plays in growth in JRA. Practical functions such as use of IGF levels to monitor growth in JRA and therapeutic trials may ensue from this knowledge.

SUMMARY AND CONCLUSIONS

Although growth retardation continues to be among the deleterious effects of JRA, the prevalence and severity in recent years appears to be decreasing. This may be due in part to disease control with early and widespread use of immunosuppressive drugs, specifically methotrexate. Another result of 'dismantling the pyramid',[63] is the decreased use of corticosteroids, perhaps the most potent of growth-suppressing agents.

Short stature continues to be strongly associated with systemic onset of disease and corticosteroid therapy. Other causative factors of growth failure include disease activity, by means of the inflammatory process and malnutrition, which may be related to decreased dietary intake from anorexia, medications and arthritis.

The role of GH and growth factor deficiencies remains less clear. Most patients have normal levels of GH. However, a subset of patients have GH deficiency and an even greater proportion of patients have low levels of IGF-1. Furthermore, the height velocity of many patients is increased, at least in the short term, by use of exogenous GH. While low levels of IGF-1 may represent a defective peripheral response to GH or the effects of malnutrition, they also may represent a relative deficiency in GH, overcome by exogenous administration of GH.

While future elucidation of the pathogenesis of growth failure is needed, much may be learned by means of well-planned intervention studies with long-term follow-up. Studies that demonstrate a reduction in the prevalence of growth failure by aggressive disease control, early nutritional support, and supplementation of GH or IGF-1, may precede our ability to answer in full why some children with JRA are small.

ACKNOWLEDGMENT

This work was supported in part by the Children's Hospital Research Foundation of Cincinnati, the Schmidlapp Foundation, the National Institutes of Health (AR42632 and AR44059) and the National Arthritis Foundation.

REFERENCES

1. Kuhns JG, Swaim LT. Disturbances of growth in chronic arthritis in children. *Am J Dis Child* 1932; **43**:1118–33.
2. Stoeber E. Prognosis in juvenile chronic arthritis. Follow-up of 433 chronic rheumatic children. *Eur J Pediatr* 1981; **135**:225–8.
3. Still GF. On a form of chronic joint disease in children. *Trans R Med Chir Soc* 1897; **80**:1–13 [reprinted in *Am J Dis Child* 1978; **132**:195–200].
4. Cassidy JT, Petty RE. *Textbook of Pediatric Rheumatology*, 3rd edn. WB Saunders: Philadelphia, 1995:135.
5. Towner SR, Michet CJ Jr, O'Fallon WM, Nelson AM. The epidemiology of juvenile rheumatoid arthritis in Rochester, Minnesota. *Arthritis Rheum* 1983; **26**:1208–13.
6. US Bureau of the Census. *Statistical Abstract of the United States*, 115th edn. Washington DC, 1995:15.
7. Ansell BM, Bywaters EGL. Growth in Still's disease. *Ann Rheum Dis* 1956; **15**:295–318.
8. Bernstein BH, Stobie D, Singsen BH, Koster-King K, Kornreich HK, Hanson V, Growth retardation in juvenile rheumatoid arthritis (JRA). *Arthritis Rheum* 1977; **20**:212–16.
9. Bacon MC, White PH, Raiten DJ et al. Nutritional status and growth in juvenile rheumatoid arthritis. *Semin Arthritis Rheum* 1990; **20**:97–106.
10. Svantesson H, Akesson A, Eberhardt K, Elborgh R. Prognosis in juvenile rheumatoid arthritis with systemic onset. *Scand J Rheumatol* 1983; **12**:139–44.
11. Fraser PA, Hoch S, Erlandson D, Partridge R, Jackson JM. The timing of menarche in juvenile rheumatoid arthritis. *J Adolesc Health Care* 1988; **9**:483–7.
12. Johansson U, Portinsson S, Akesson A, Svantesson H, Ockerman PA, Akesson B. Nutritional status of girls with juvenile chronic arthritis. *Hum Nutr Clin Nutr* 1986; **40c**:57–67.
13. Lovell DJ, White PH. Growth and nutrition in juvenile rheumatoid arthritis. In: *Paediatric Rheumatology Update* (Woo P, White P, Ansell B, eds.). Oxford University Press: Oxford, 1990:47–56.
14. Gare BA, Fasth A. The natural history of juvenile chronic arthritis: a population based cohort study. II. Outcome. *J Rheumatol* 1995; **22**:308–19.
15. Hamill PVV, Drizd TA, Johnson CL, Reed RB, Roche AF, Moore WM. Physical growth: National Center for Health Statistics percentiles. *Am J Clin Nutr* 1979; **32**:607–29.
16. Cameron N. The methods of auxological anthropometry. In: *Human Growth – A Comprehensive Treatise*, vol 3 (Falkner F, Tanner JM, eds.). New York: Plenum Press, 1986:3–46.
17. Svantesson H, Marhaug G, Haeffner F. Scoliosis in children with juvenile rheumatoid arthritis. *Scand J Rheumatology* 1981; **10**:65–8.
18. Simon S, Whiffen J, Shapiro F. Leg length discrepancies in monarticular and pauciarticular juvenile rheumatoid arthritis. *J Bone Joint Surg* 1981; **63A**:209–15.
19. Lovell DJ, Woo P. Growth and skeletal maturation. In: *Oxford Textbook of Rheumatology* (Maddison PJ, Isenberg DA, Woo P, Glass DN eds.). Oxford University Press: Oxford, 1993;481–96.
20. Martini A, Ravelli A, Notarangelo LD et al. Enhanced interleukin 1 and depressed interleukin 2 production in juvenile arthritis. *J Rheumatol* 1986; **13**:598–603.
21. Haugen MA, Hoyeraal HM, Larsen S, Gilboe IM, Trygg K. Nutrient intake and nutritional status in children with juvenile chronic arthritis. *Scand J Rheumatol* 1992; **21**:165–70.

22. Hintz RL, Suskind R, Amatayakul K, Thanangkul O, Olsen R. Plasma somatomedin and growth hormone values in children with protein–calorie malnutrition. *J Pediatr* 1978; **92**:153–6.
23. Clemmons DR, Underwood LE. Nutritional regulation of IGF-1 and IGF binding proteins. *Ann Rev Nutr* 1991; **11**:393–412.
24. Laaksonen AL. A prognostic study of juvenile rheumatoid arthritis: analysis of 544 cases. *Acta Paed Scand* 1966; **166** (Suppl):49–55.
25. Hunt PG, Vinton NE, Ross CD. Height velocity with methotrexate therapy in juvenile rheumatoid arthritis [abstract]. *Arthritis Rheum* 1994; **37** (Suppl):S276.
26. Coss JA, Boots RH. Juvenile rheumatoid arthritis. A study of fifty-six cases with a note on skeletal changes. *J Pediatr* 1946; **29**:143–56.
27. Lockie LM, Norcross BM. Juvenile rheumatoid arthritis. *Pediatrics* 1948; **2**:694–8.
28. Mascioli EA, Blackburn GL. Nutrition and rheumatic diseases. In: *Textbook of Rheumatology* (Kelly WN, Harris ED, Ruddy S, Sledge CB, eds.). WB Saunders: Philadelphia, 1985:352–60.
29. Lovell DJ, Gregg D, Heubi J, Levinson JE. Nutritional status in juvenile rheumatoid arthritis (JRA) – an interim report [abstract]. *J Rheumatol* 1983; **13**:979.
30. Warady BD, McCamman SP, Lindsley CB. Anthropometric assessment of patients with juvenile rheumatoid arthritis. *Top Clin Nutr* 1989; **4**:7–14.
31. Henderson CJ, Lovell DJ. Assessment of protein–energy malnutrition in children and adolescents with juvenile rheumatoid arthritis. *Arthritis Care Res* 1989; **2**:108–13.
32. Henderson CJ, Lovell DJ, Gregg DJ. A nutritional screening test for use in children and adolescents with juvenile rheumatoid arthritis. *J Rheumatol* 1992; **19**:1276–81.
33. Miller ML, Chacko JA, Young EA. Dietary deficiencies in children with juvenile rheumatoid arthritis. *Arthritis Care Res* 1989; **2**:22–4.
34. Mortensen AL, Allen JR, Allen RC. Nutritional assessment of children with juvenile chronic arthritis. *J Paediatr Child Health* 1990; **26**:335–8.
35. Larheim TA, Hoyeraal HM, Stabrun AE et al. The temporomandibular joint in juvenile rheumatoid arthritis. Radiographic changes related to clinical and laboratory parameters in 100 children. *Scand J Rheumatol* 1982; **11**:5–12.
36. Lovell D, Henderson C. Juvenile rheumatoid arthritis. In: *Pediatric Nutrition in Chronic Diseases and Developmental Disorders* (Ekvall SW, ed.). Oxford University Press: New York, 1993:263–8.
37. Blodgett FM, Burgin L, Iezzoni D, Gribetz D, Talbot NB. Effects of prolonged cortisone therapy on the statural growth, skeletal maturation and metabolic status of children. *N Engl J Med* 1956; **254**:636–41.
38. Van Metre TE Jr, Niermann WA, Rosen LJ. A comparison of the growth suppressive effect of cortisone, prednisone, and other adrenal cortical hormones. *J Allergy* 1960; **31**:531–42.
39. Hyams JS, Carey DE. Corticosteroids and growth. *J Pediatr* 1988; **113**:249–54.
40. Zutshi DW, Friedman M, Ansell BM. Corticotrophin therapy in juvenile chronic polyarthritis (Still's disease) and effect on growth. *Arch Dis Child* 1971; **46**:584–93.
41. Sturge RA, Beardwell C, Hartog M, Wright D, Ansell BM. Cortisol and growth hormone secretion in relation to linear growth: patients with Still's disease on different therapeutic regiments. *Br Med J* 1970; **3**:547–51.
42. Loftus J, Allen R, Hesp R et al. Randomized, double-blind trial of deflazacort versus prednisone in juvenile chronic (or rheumatoid) arthritis: a relatively bone-sparing effect of deflazacort. *Pediatrics* 1991; **88**:428–36.
43. Ferraris JR, Pasqualini T. Therapy with a new glucocorticoid: effect of deflazacort on linear growth and growth hormone secretion in renal transplantation. *J Rheumatol* 1993; **20** (Suppl 37):43–6.
44. Ansell BA, Bywaters EGL. Alternate-day corticosteroid therapy in juvenile chronic polyarthritis. *J Rheumatol* 1974; **1**:176–86.
45. Byron MA, Jackson J, Ansell BM. Effect of different corticosteroid regimens on hypothalamic–pituitary axis and growth in juvenile chronic arthritis. *J R Soc Med* 1983; **76**:452–7.
46. Elders MJ, Wingfield BS, McNatt ML, Clarke JS, Hughes ER. Glucocorticoid therapy in children: effect on somatomedin secretion. *Am J Dis Child* 1975; **129**:1393–6.
47. Richards GE, Pachman LM, Green OC. Symptomatic hypothyroidism in children with collagen disease. *J Pediatr* 1975; **87**:82–4.
48. Yarom A, Rennenbohm RM, Levinson JE. Antithyroid antibody (ATA) positivity in juvenile rheumatoid arthritis [abstract]. *Clin Res* 1984; **32**:793A.

49. Rallison ML, Dobyns BM, Keating FR, Rall JE, Tyler FH. Occurrence and natural history of chronic lymphocytic thyroiditis in childhood. *J Pediatr* 1975; **86**:675–82.
50. Butenandt O. Rheumatoid arthritis and growth retardation in children: treatment with human growth hormone. *Eur J Pediatr* 1979; **130**:15–28.
51. Chipman JJ, Boyar RM, Fink CW. Anterior-pituitary adrenal function of gold–treated patients with juvenile rheumatoid arthritis. *J Rheumatol* 1982; **9**:63–8.
52. Falcini F, Taccetti G, Trapani S, Tafi L, Volpi M. Growth retardation in juvenile chronic arthritis patients treated with steroids. *Clin Exp Rheumatol* 1991; **9** (Suppl 6):37–40.
53. Allen RC, Jimenez M, Cowell CT. Insulin-like growth factor and growth hormone secretion in juvenile chronic arthritis. *Ann Rheum Dis* 1991; **50**:602–6.
54. Davies UM, Rooney M, Preece MA, Ansell BA, Woo P. Treatment of growth retardation in juvenile chronic arthritis with recombinant human growth hormone. *J Rheumatol* 1994; **21**:153–8.
55. Hopp RJ, Degan J, Corley K, Lindsley CB, Cassidy JT. Evaluation of growth hormone secretion in children with JRA and short stature. *Nebr Med J* 1995; **80**:52–7.
56. Kammerer WH, Stokes PE. Effects of human growth hormone in a girl dwarfed from rheumatoid arthritis and corticosteroid therapy. *Arthritis Rheum* 1962; **5**:304–5.
57. Ward DJ, Hartog M, Ansell BM. Corticosteroid-induced dwarfism in Still's disease treated with human growth hormone. Clinical and metabolic effects including hydroxyproline excretion in two cases. *Ann Rheum Dis* 1966; **26**:416–21.
58. Svantesson H. Treatment of growth failure with human growth hormone in patients with juvenile chronic arthritis. A pilot study. *Clin Exp Rheumatol* 1991; **9** (Suppl 6):47–50.
59. Rivkees SA, Danon M, Herrin J. Prednisone dose limitation of growth hormone treatment of steroid-induced growth failure. *J Pediatr* 1994; **125**:322–5.
60. Martha PM, Reiter EO. Pubertal growth and growth hormone secretion. *Endocrinol Metab Clin North Am* 1991; **20**:165–82.
61. Bennett AE, Silverman ED, Miller JJ, Hintz RL. Insulin-like growth factors I and II in children with systemic onset juvenile arthritis. *J Rheumatol* 1988; **15**:655–8.
62. Aitman TJ, Palmer RG, Loftus J et al. Serum IGF-I levels and growth failure in juvenile chronic arthritis. *Clin Exp Rheumatol* 1989; **7**:557–61.
63. Levinson JE, Wallace CA. Dismantling the pyramid. *J Rheumatol* 1992; **19** (Suppl 33):6–10.

15

Is the treatment of autoimmune rheumatic diseases the same in children as in adults?

Lori B Tucker

The spectrum of rheumatic diseases occurring in childhood includes most of the common rheumatic diseases of adulthood, such as chronic arthritis, systemic lupus erythematosus (SLE), dermatomyositis, scleroderma, and the vasculitides. There are similarities in pathophysiological findings in rheumatic diseases seen in children and adults. The histopathology of chronic synovitis of rheumatoid arthritis (RA) and juvenile RA (JRA) is similar. Childhood-onset and adult-onset SLE are both characterized by a similar spectrum of serum autoantibodies and immune-complex-mediated organ system damage.

Despite these similarities, however, there are significant differences in the types and frequencies of diseases seen, their clinical presentations, and course, in paediatric patients. Some of the most striking differences can be seen in the types of arthritis seen in children vs those seen most commonly in adults. There are five types of chronic inflammatory arthritis seen in childhood (these are further reviewed in Chapter 12). The paediatric 'equivalent' of adult RA, seropositive polyarticular JRA, is the least common subtype of JRA seen in paediatric rheumatology clinics,[1] whereas the most common subtype of JRA, pauciarticular disease, has no true adult-onset counterpart. Systemic-onset JRA, previously known as Still's disease, is seen in approximately 15% of the JRA population,[1] but is much less common in adults. Other common adult rheumatic disorders, such as osteoarthritis and gout, are very rarely seen in the paediatric rheumatology clinic. Systemic lupus presenting in childhood tends to be more severe at presentation than adult-onset disease, and the prevalence of clinical features varies.[2] Dermatomyositis is by far the most common idiopathic inflammatory myopathy seen in childhood, with polymyositis more common in adult populations.[3] Linear scleroderma is seen more commonly in children than adults. The most common vasculitides of childhood, Kawasaki disease and Henoch Schönlein purpura, are relatively rare in adulthood.

Against this background of clinically differing diseases with seemingly similar underlying pathophysiology, it is of interest to speculate about the treatment of rheumatic conditions in children and adults and whether these diseases require different approaches. In this review, current therapeutic approaches to the major autoimmune rheumatic conditions of childhood – chronic arthritis, SLE, and dermatomyositis – will be reviewed and compared to treatment protocols used in adult patients. I hope to convince the reader that, in fact, children are not merely miniature adults when it comes to the treatment of rheumatic disorders!

JUVENILE RHEUMATOID ARTHRITIS

Decision making in the treatment of JRA must include an understanding of the subtype of the disease and its course in any individual patient.

JRA is divided into three major onset subtypes, assigned by the patient's presentation within 6 months of disease onset.[4] Terminology and classification of chronic arthritis in childhood is controversial, with the term JRA used in North America and JCA (juvenile chronic arthritis) used in Europe. A further review of these controversies can be found in Chapter 12. In this chapter, I will use the term 'JRA' throughout to refer to chronic arthritis in childhood.

The subtypes of JRA are: systemic-onset, polyarticular, and pauciarticular-onset. Assignment of disease subtype is not a mere matter of semantics; clinical features, response to medication, and outcomes differ among JRA subtypes. Systemic-onset JRA accounts for approximately 15% of children with JRA, and presents with predominant extra-articular features such as daily spiking fevers, characteristic rash, lymphadenopathy, hepatosplenomegaly, and elevated acute-phase reactants. Arthritis may not be an important clinical feature early in disease presentation, but a significant percentage of children with systemic-onset JRA develop severe, persistent, and erosive joint disease over time. Most children with polyarticular JRA (more than five joints involved) are seronegative for rheumatoid factor. These children, generally young girls, may develop significant joint erosions and disability over years. A small subgroup of children with polyarticular disease are positive for rheumatoid factor, and these children have disease which more closely resembles adult-onset RA in course and therefore require more aggressive early treatment. The most common subtype of JRA is pauciarticular disease (fewer than four joints involved), occurring most frequently in young girls; generally with monoarticular disease involving the knee. There is no adult equivalent of this subtype of JRA. The prognosis for most children with pauciarticular JRA is very good, with a significant percentage of children entering remission during childhood. However, perhaps up to 15% of children with pauciarticular-onset disease may progress to a polyarticular course at some point during their disease course, and it is believed generally that this portends a poorer outcome. In addition, 25–30% of children with pauciarticular-onset JRA will develop subacute anterior uveitis which can lead to permanent visual damage if undetected or inadequately treated.[5]

Table 15.1 Drug therapy for juvenile rheumatoid arthritis

Nonsteroidal anti-inflammatory agents
Naproxen
Tolmetin
Ibuprofen
Indomethacin
Others less commonly prescribed
Sulphasalazine
Injectable gold
Methotrexate – oral or injectable
Corticosteroids – oral, intravenous, or intra-articular
Newer agents
Intravenous immunoglobulin
Cyclosporin

Despite the significant differences among the various subtypes and disease courses in JRA, one can make general comments about the drug therapy of arthritis in children in comparison to adults. The therapeutic pyramid of initial treatment with nonsteroidal anti-inflammatory drugs (NSAIDs) followed by more aggressive second-line drugs and immunosuppressants is used as a paradigm by most paediatric rheumatologists (Table 15.1). Recently, this approach has been called into question in paediatric rheumatology, as it has been in adult rheumatology, with some calling for earlier aggressive treatment for children in whom one can predict the potential for a poor outcome.[5–8]

Nearly all children with JRA require treatment with NSAIDs at some point in the course of their disease. The choice of NSAIDs to use in paediatrics is limited, in that most agents have not undergone study in children, and in the USA, few NSAIDs have approval for use in paediatrics. Aspirin, an old standby in the treatment of JRA, is much less in favour, due to relatively common side-effects such as hepatotoxicity, the need for frequent dosing, and the risk of Reye's syndrome. The most frequently used NSAIDs in children with JRA are naproxen, tolmetin, ibuprofen, and indomethacin, with fewer children prescibed the myriad of newer agents available over recent years. The popular NSAIDs have known dosing schedules and convenient dosage preparations, such as liquid, for children.[9,10]. Newer drugs are often not appropriate, due to unknown dosing schedules for small children and unavailability of dosing formats that children can take. There have been few comparative studies in paediatrics to establish relative effectiveness of NSAIDs in the treatment of JRA.

Although many of the same drugs are used in children as in adults with RA, the side-effects differ. Gastrointestinal toxicity such as gastritis and ulcers is well documented as a common occurrence in adults taking NSAIDs.[11] There have been relatively few studies that have examined the occurrence of gastrointestinal toxicity of NSAIDs in children with JRA.[12–14] Mulberg et al[12] found gastritis, antral erosions, or ulcers in 75% of a group of 17 children with JRA treated with NSAIDs, and referred to the paediatric gastroenterologist for evaluation of abdominal pain or an unexpected drop in haematocrit. Hermaszewski et al[14] found fewer and milder abnormalities by endoscopy in a similar group of 13 children with JRA taking NSAIDs. Keenan et al[13] performed a retrospective review of computer records of children with JRA being followed in a single clinic, and identified only five children with defined 'significant gastropathy'. From these studies, one might conclude that significant gastrointestinal complications of NSAID therapy may be less common among children with JRA. However, the studies are limited by small sample size, and identification of patients only by reported symptoms or retrospective review. The true incidence of gastrointestinal complications of NSAIDs in children is unknown, and further studies need to be carried out.

In 1990, paediatric rheumatology centres began to report an unusually high occurrence of a previously rarely reported side-effect of NSAIDs, 'pseudoporphyria'.[15,16] This skin problem, manifested by small bullous vesicular eruptions in sun-exposed areas, increased skin fragility, and the development of characteristic pitted scars had been known occur, although rarely, with exposure to NSAIDs, particularly naproxen. Wallace et al[17] reported facial scars from pseudoporphyria in 9% of a population of 250 children with JRA taking NSAIDs, with lesions found in 22% of children taking naproxen. Children with fair skin and blue or green eyes appear to be more susceptible to this particular photosensitivity reaction. Children using naproxen had a relative risk of 6.0 for development of pseudoporphyria, a much higher rate than reported in the drug information. The facial scars of pseudoporphyria heal, but slowly, over a long period of time. Similar high frequencies of pseudoporphyria have not been reported from adult rheumatology clinics, and it may be concluded that this side-effect is more prevalent among children.

The indications for the use of second-line agents in children with JRA are as unclear as the indications in adult arthritis; that is, there are no published specific guidelines that suggest which patients best benefit or at what point in the disease course a second-line agent should be added.[18] Although the armamentarium of medications is similar in children compared to adults, there are clear differences in choices and efficacy in paediatrics. For example, studies have not shown hydroxychloroquine or penicillamine to be more effective than placebo for the treatment of JRA,[19] and therefore they are not popular medication choices of paediatric rheumatologists. Sulphasalazine as a low toxicity, intermediate-action second-line agent has variable use in adult and paediatric rheumatology. Some adult rheumatology clinics report using sulphasalazine early in the course of RA in the hope of preventing aggressive disease.[6,20] There have been several small open trials of sulphasalazine in children with JRA, with beneficial results in children with spondyloarthropathy.[21,22] There have been anecdotal reports of an increase in serious toxic reactions in children with systemic JRA,[23] and therefore caution should be used in prescribing this drug to these children. Prior to the advent of the 'age of methotrexate', injectable gold was a common therapy for childhood arthritis. Retrospective studies report improvement rates ranging from 18% to 78%,[19,23] making accurate assessment of the efficacy of this drug difficult. However, it is the only drug for which remission rates have been reported, making it attractive as a choice for children who fail methotrexate therapy. One important difference in the use of gold in children with JRA is that serious toxicity, including death, have been reported in children with active systemic JRA given gold injections.[24,25] Many paediatric rheumatologists feel gold is contraindicated in this group of children. The common mode of administration of gold (injections!) is disliked by children and parents universally. With an attractive alternative choice such as methotrexate available, this has led to a decline in the use of injectable gold in the paediatric rheumatology clinic.

Methrotrexate is the most frequently used second-line agent used for treating JRA, as it is in adults with RA.[26] A recent meta-analysis of drug trials in JRA showed methotrexate to be the most effective agent among those which have been tested to date.[19,27] The safety profile of methotrexate in children is as good as in adult patients, and studies following children for 5 years and longer have not shown any significant long-term concerns.[28–30] Recent studies have suggested that children tolerate higher doses of methotrexate than do adults, and Wallace et al have shown in a small series that children with an inadequate response to standard doses of methotrexate (10 mg/m^2 per week) showed a good response to higher doses, up to 1 mg/kg per week (doses equivalent to 15–20 mg/m^2 per week).[31]

Steroid therapy for children with JRA is utilized in a very different manner from the way it is prescribed for adults with RA. Low-dose daily steroid therapy, a common, if controversial, approach in the treatment of adult RA, is rarely indicated for children with JRA.[5,18,32] The short-term side-effects of unnecessary weight gain and increased susceptibility to infection cause difficulties for children, and the longer-term side-effect of growth suppression is particularly devastating for those who already may have difficulty with growth because of their disease. Steroids in high doses may be necessary for children with systemic-onset JRA who have severe systemic complications such as anaemia or pericarditis, or whose fever is not responsive to NSAIDs.[32] Intra-articular steroid therapy is a useful management technique for children with persistent disease in selected joints, and recent studies have shown this form of therapy to be safe in childhood.[33]

Some children with JRA have resistant, persistently active disease, despite the best efforts with all of the above treatments. There have been encouraging reports of the use of cyclosporin in these children,[34] with considerable improvement in a small study of nine children with either systemic-onset or polyarticular disease poorly responsive to standard therapies.[35] The side-effects of cyclosporin are considerable, but further studies should certainly be carried out in larger patient groups.

Intravenous immunoglobulin (IVIG) in high doses has also been proposed as a novel treatment for recalcitrant JRA; however, a recent multicentre trial did not show substantial benefit of IVIG administered to children with refractory systemic-onset JRA.[36]

Physical and occupational therapy play a critical role in the rehabilitation of children with JRA. A complete discussion of physical rehabilitation of JRA is beyond the scope of this chapter; however, it is important for rehabilitation protocols to be designed and undertaken with an understanding of the disease processes, childhood development, and family involvement.[37] Programmes focused purely on joint flexibility are inadequate, as attention needs to be paid to functional assessment and developmental achievement. Children with JRA should be evaluated by therapists with experience in paediatric rheumatology, who can prescribe a therapeutic exercise programme, suggest modifications for school, encourage compliance, and teach the family how best to help their child with arthritis.[38] Participation in school and community activities are critical for normal child development; there is no longer any excuse for children with JRA or other rheumatic conditions to be excused from school for long periods of time. Rheumatologists and therapists must work together with families to devise creative solutions to maintain children with JRA in regular school programming.[38,39]

DERMATOMYOSITIS

In childhood, dermatomyositis is the most common of the idiopathic inflammatory myositis disorders seen, and therefore this discussion will be focused on its treatment. Dermatomyositis was known to be a disease with a poor outcome in the presteroid era, with up to 30% mortality reported.[40,41] One of the very first reports of the successful treatment of dermatomyositis with corticosteroids was in a group of paediatric patients with the condition.[42] Since that time, the efficacy of corticosteroids in the treatment of dermatomyositis has become well established, although there have been no attempts at placebo-controlled treatment trials to substantiate this. In general, steroid treatment protocols used in paediatric patients and adult patients with dermatomyositis are similar.[43] Most rheumatologists would agree with the philosophy of initiation of therapy with high doses of corticosteroids, maintained until serum muscle enzymes are normal and muscle strength is improving, and slow tapering of therapy while the possibility of disease flares is monitored. However, corticosteroid dosing in paediatrics is calculated on a weight basis, with most paediatric rheumatologists suggesting initiating therapy with doses of approximately 2 mg/kg per day, as compared with suggested doses of 40–80 mg/day for larger adult patients.[44] High-dose intravenous pulse corticosteroids have been advocated by some paediatric rheumatologists as an attempt at aggressive disease treatment and sparing of significant steroid-related side-effects.[45] However, there have been no comparison studies to determine which mode of therapy is best, oral or intravenous.

Patients with dermatomyositis whose disease responds incompletely to steroid therapy, or who develop intolerable steroid side-effects, or who develop disease flares as the steroid dose is tapered, are candidates for treatment with immunosuppressive agents. The immunosuppressive agents used for dermatomyositis include azathioprine, methotrexate, cyclosporin, and cyclophosphamide.[3,46] Because there have never been adequate randomized treatment trials to compare the efficacy of these drugs, the choice of the best drug to use is often anecdotal and dependent on individual rheumatologist's comfort and experience. In juvenile dermatomyositis, there have been several reports that have shown the efficacy and safety of methotrexate as a second-line immunosuppressive agent.[47] Azathioprine, often suggested as a second-line agent for adult recalcitrant dermatomyositis, is less commonly used in juvenile dermatomyositis.[3,44] Cyclosporin as a second-line immunospressive for dermatomyositis was reported first in paediatric patients, and there are now a number of reports that show efficacy for children with disease unresponsive to methotrexate or azathioprine.[48]

All of the immunosuppressive agents used in the treatment of dermatomyositis have significant toxicities, which may limit their benefits. Recently, attempts to identify an alternative therapeutic agent for myositis led to trials of high-dose IVIG, with promising results.[49] Although the majority of the reported cases are adults with polymyositis or dermatomyositis, there have been a number of small series of children with dermatomyositis reported as showing improvement with IVIG therapy[50–53] (Table 15.2). These studies have reported effective control of dermatomyositis in children whose disease was recalcitrant to treatment with immunosuppressive agents or in whom intolerable steroid side-effects developed. In

Table 15.2 Treatment of juvenile dermatomyositis with intravenous immunoglobulin: a review of the literature

Reference	Number of patients	Age (years)	Number of cycles[a]	Improvements[b]			
				Muscle strength	Rash	Muscle enzymes	Tapering steroids
Roifman et al[53]	1	15	6	100	NR	75	100
Lang et al[50]	5	2.5–15	9	80	100	50	100
Collet et al[52]	2	7, 12	9	100	100	100	100
Sansome and Dubowitz[51]	9	10.6[c]	mean 4	80	NR	NR	25

[a]Number of monthly treatments with intravenonus immunoglobulin.
[b]Results are % of patients improved.
[c]Mean age.
NR = not recorded

particular, IVIG appears to be effective in treating severe skin disease, which is frequently recalcitrant to other therapies. Therefore, this new application of an old treatment modality appears to be equally effective in the paediatric and the adult populations.

SYSTEMIC LUPUS ERYTHEMATOSUS

Prescription of effective therapy for patients with SLE is a challenge, requiring careful and long-term evaluation of clinical symptoms and laboratory markers, as well as patient well-being and functional abilities. The standard therapeutic regimens for adults with SLE are well described.[54] In general, NSAIDs and hydroxychloroquine are sufficient for patients with mild skin, joint, or other minor clinical manifestations of disease. Patients with major organ system disease, such as nephritis, serositis, or disease flares, often require steroid treatment, and the addition of cytotoxic agents such as azathioprine and cyclophosphamide is reserved generally for patients with severe organ system disease flares or unacceptable steroid toxicity. There is controversy concerning the most effective steroid dosing schedules and methods of administration (intravenous pulses, oral, alternate day oral therapy), as well as when to begin cytotoxic therapies.[55]

The basic principles of treatment for SLE outlined above are similar for childhood-onset SLE. Children with SLE seem to have more severe disease onset than adults,[2] and therefore may be treated with steroids more frequently in higher doses (Table 15.1). There has never been a randomized controlled trial of treatment regimens or even a large-scale treatment trial in childhood SLE; therefore, paediatric rheumatologists apply outcome data from adult studies to their paediatric patients. Interpretation of treatment outcomes in paediatric SLE are hampered by the smaller numbers of patients per centre.

Significant disagreements exist among paediatric rheumatologists concerning the best cytotoxic agent to use in children with SLE: azathioprine or cyclophosphamide.[56,57] Some clinicians report good success in treating renal disease in childhood SLE with cyclophosphamide,[58] and strongly recommend this course of therapy for all children with SLE and renal disease. Others[57] equally forcefully favour the use of azathioprine for this indication. Comparative studies have not been done.

Therapies for SLE other than the above-described standard treatments have been reported even more rarely in children. Methotrexate has been reported to be effective in several small series of adult patients with SLE;[59,60] the first series reported, however, was a group of 10 children with SLE treated with low-dose oral weekly methotrexate in whom a significant prednisone- or cytoxtoxic-sparing effect was seen.[61]

SLE is a chronic disease which invariably affects the psychological and functional development of affected children in ways quite different from those in their adult counterparts. The majority of affected children with SLE are in the adolescent age range, a time when the normal development tasks of developing independence from family and a healthy body and sexual image is considerably impacted by the presence of a serious chronic illness such as SLE. Difficulty in accepting the diagnosis, depression, anger at being 'different' from peers, and risk-taking behaviour such as not taking medications are all very common in adolescents with SLE, and physicians caring for such patients need to anticipate these problems and provide guidance and support for these patients and their families. School participation is the childhood equivalent of work, and full continuous school participation should be the goal of every child with SLE. Care of the total child with SLE and their family is a challenge; in this instance, it must be emphasized that children with SLE are not just 'small adults'!

CONCLUSION

What can we conclude from this discussion about the therapy of childhood rheumatic conditions? Are there significant differences from the therapy of adult rheumatic diseases? Although there are certainly many similarities in the drugs used in children and adults, I believe the bulk of evidence and experience of paediatric rheumatologists leads to the conclusion that childhood rheumatic conditions have many unique characteristics, and therapy for these diseases of childhood requires special understanding, expertise, and experience in the area of paediatrics. Children with rheumatic conditions offer special challenges with respect to changing developmental levels, different responses to medications, and family involvement in care.

REFERENCES

1. DeNardo BA, Tucker LB, Miller LC, Szer IS, Schaller JG. Demography of a regional paediatric rheumatology patient population. *J Rheum* 1994; **21**:1553–61.
2. Tucker LB, Menon S, Schaller JG, Isenberg DA. Adult- and childhood-onset systemic lupus erythematosus: A comparison of onset, clinical features, serology, and outcome. *Br J Rheum* 1995; **34**:866–72.
3. Dalakas MC. Clinical, immunopathologic, and therapeutic considerations of inflammatory myopathies. *Clin Neuropharmacol* 1992; **15**:327–51.
4. Cassidy JT, Levinson JE, Brewer EJ. The development of classification criteria for children with juvenile rheumatoid arthritis. *Bull Rheum Dis* 1989; **38**:1–7.
5. Schaller JG. Therapy for childhood rheumatic diseases. *Arthritis Rheum* 1993; **36**:65–70.
6. Emery P. Therapeutic approaches for early rheumatoid arthritis. How early? How aggressive? *Br J Rheum* 1995; **34** (Suppl 2):87–90.
7. Levinson JE, Wallace C. Dismantling the pyramid. *J Rheum* 1992; **33** (Suppl):6–10.
8. Wilske KR, Healey LA. Challenging the therapeutic pyramid: a new look at treatment strategies for rheumatoid arthritis. *J Rheum* 1990; **25** (Suppl):4–7.
9. Giannini EH, Brewer EJ, Miller ML, Gibbas D, Passo MH, Hoyerall HM, Bernstein B, Person DA, Fink CW, Sawyer LA, Scheinbaum ML. Ibuprofen suspension in the treatment of juvenile rheumatoid arthritis. *J Pediatr* 1990; **117**:645–52.

10. Levinson JE, Baum J, Brewer EJ, Fink C, Hanson V, Schaller JG. Comparison of tolmetin sodium and aspirin in the treatment of juvenile rheumatoid arthritis. *J Pediatr* 1977; **91**:799–804.
11. Simon LS. Actions and toxic effects of nonsteroidal anti-inflammatory drugs. *Current Opin Rheum* 1994; **6**:238–51.
12. Mulberg AE, Linz C, Bern E, Tucker L, Verhave M, Grand RJ. Identification of nonsteroidal antiinflammatory drug-induced gastroduodenal injury in children with juvenile rheumatoid arthritis. *J Pediatr* 1993; **122**:647–9.
13. Keenan GF, Giannini EH, Athreya BH. Clinically significant gastropathy associated with nonsteroidal antiinflammatory drug use in children with juvenile rheumatoid arthritis. *J Rheum* 1995; **22**:1149–51.
14. Hermaszewski R, Hayllar J, Woo P. Gastroduodenal damage due to nonsteroidal anti-inflammatory drugs in children. *Br J Rheum* 1993; **32**:69–72.
15. Allen R, Rogers M, Humphrey I. Naproxen induced pseudoporphyria in juvenile chronic arthritis. *J Rheum* 1991; **18**:893–6.
16. Levy ML, Barron KS, Eichenfield A, Honig PJ. Naproxen-induced pseudoporphyria: A distinctive photodermatitis. *J Pediatr* 1990; **117**:660–4.
17. Wallace CA, Farrow D, Sherry DD. Increased risk of facial scars in children taking non-steroidal antiinflammatory drugs. *J Pediatr* 1994; **125**:819–22.
18. Athreya BH, Cassidy JT. Current status of the medical treatment of children with juvenile rheumatoid arthritis. *Rheum Dis Clin North Am* 1991; **17**:871–89.
19. Giannini EH, Cassidy JT, Brewer EJ, Shaikov A, Maximov A, Kuzmina N. Comparative efficacy and safety of advanced drug therapy in children with juvenile rheumatoid arthritis. *Semin Arthritis Rheum* 1993; **23**:34–46.
20. Van Riel PLCM, Van Gestel AM, Van De Putte LBA. Long-term usage and side-effect profile of sulphasalazine in rheumatoid arthritis. *Br J Rheum* 1995; **34** (Suppl 2):40–2.
21. Joos R, Veys EM, Mielants H, van Werveke S, Goemaere S. Sulfasalazine treatment in juvenile chronic arthritis: An open study. *J Rheum* 1991; **18**:880–4.
22. Rosenberg AM. Advanced drug therapy for juvenile rheumatoid arthritis. *J Pediatr* 1989; **114**:171–8.
23. Rooney M. Is there a disease-modifying drug for juvenile chronic arthritis? *Br J Rheum* 1992; **31**:635–641.
24. Jacobs JC, Gorin LJ, Hanissian AS, Simon JL, Smithwick EM, Sullivan D. Consumption coagulopathy after gold therapy for juvenile rheumatoid arthritis [letter]. *J Pediatr* 1984; **105**:674–5.
25. Silverman ED, Miller JJ, Bernstein B, Shafai T. Consumption coagulopathy associated with systemic juvenile rheumatoid arthritis. *J Pediatr* 1983; **103**:872–6.
26. Weinblatt ME. Efficacy of methotrexate in rheumatoid arthritis. *Br J Rheum* 1995; **34** (Suppl 2):43–8.
27. Giannini EH, Brewer EJ, Kuzima N, Shaikov A, Maximov A, Voronstov I, Fink CW, Newman AJ, Cassidy JT, Zemel LS. Methotrexate in resistant juvenile rheumatoid arthritis: Results of the USA–USSR double-blind, placebo-controlled trial. *N Engl J Med* 1992; **326**:1043–9.
28. Graham LD, Myones BL, Rivas-Chacon RF, Pachman LM. Morbidity associated with long-term methotrexate therapy in juvenile rheumatoid arthritis. *J Pediatr* 1992; **120**:468–73.
29. Rose CD, Singsen BH, Eichenfield AH, Goldsmith DP, Athreya BH. Safety and efficacy of methotrexate therapy for juvenile rheumatoid arthritis. *J Pediatr* 1990; **117**:653–9.
30. Kugathasan S, Newman AJ, Dahms BB, Boyle JT. Liver biopsy findings in patients with juvenile rheumatoid arthritis receiving long-term, weekly methotrexate therapy. *J Pediatr* 1996; **128**:149–51.
31. Wallace CA, Sherry DD. Preliminary report of higher dose methotrexate treatment in juvenile rheumatoid arthritis. *J Rheum* 1992; **19**:1604–7.
32. Fink CW. Overview of corticosteroid therapy in the different rheumatic diseases of childhood. *Clin Exp Rheum* 1991; **9** (Suppl 6):9–13.
33. Huppertz HI, Tschammler A, Horwitz AE, Schwab KO. Intraarticular corticosteroids for chronic arthritis in children: efficacy and effects on cartilage and growth. *J Pediatr* 1995; **127**:317–21.
34. Ansell BM. Cyclosporin A in paediatric rheumatology. *Clin Exp Rheum* 1993; **11**:113–5.
35. Pistoia V, Buoncompagni A, Scribanis R, Fasce L, Alpigiani G, Cordone G, Ferrarini M, Borrone C, Cottafava F. Cyclosporin A in the treatment of juvenile chronic arthritis and childhood polymyositis-dermatomyositis. Results of a preliminary study. *Clin Exp Rheum* 1993; **11**:203–8.
36. Silverman ED, Cawkwell GD, Lovell DJ, Laxer

RM, Lehman TJ, Passo MH, Zemel LS, Giannini EH. Intravenous immunoglobulin in the treatment of systemic juvenile rheumatoid arthritis: a randomized placebo controlled trial. Pediatric Rheumatology Collaborative Study Group. *J Rheum* 1994; **21**:2353–8.

37. Emery HM, Bowyer SL, Sisung CE. Rehabilitation of the child with a rheumatic disease. *Pediatr Clin North Am* 1995; **42**:1263–83.
38. Tucker LB, DeNardo BA, Stebulis J, Schaller JG. *Your Child with Arthritis: A Family Guide for Caregiving*. Baltimore, MD: The Johns Hopkins University Press, 1996.
39. Spencer CH, Fife RZ, Rabinovich CE. The school experience of children with arthritis. *Pediatr Clin North Am* 1995; **42**:1285–98.
40. Jacobs JC. Treatment of dermatomyositis. *Arthritis Rheum* 1977; **20**:338–41.
41. Sullivan DB, Cassidy JT, Petty RE, Burt MT. Prognosis in childhood dermatomyositis. *J Pediatr* 1972; **80**:555–63.
42. Wedgwood RJP, Cook CD, Cohen J. Dermatomyositis: Report of 26 cases in children with a discussion of endocrine therapy in 13. *Pediatrics* 1953; **12**:447–66.
43. Oddis CV, Medsger TAJ. Relationship between serum creatinine kinase level and corticosteroid level in polymyositis/dermatomyositis. *J Rheum* 1988; **15**:807–11.
44. Kaye SA, Isenberg DA. Treatment of polymyositis and dermatomyositis. *Br J Hosp Med* 1994; **52**:463–8.
45. Pachman LM. Juvenile dermatomyositis: A clinical overview. *Pediatr Rev* 1990; **12**:117–25.
46. Arnett FC, Whelton JC, Zizic TM, Stevens MB. Methotrexate therapy in polymyositis. *Ann Rheum Dis* 1973; **32**:536–46.
47. Miller LC, Sisson BA, Tucker LB, DeNardo BA, Schaller JG. Methotrexate treatment of recalcitrant childhood dermatomyositis. *Arthritis Rheum* 1992; **35**:1143–9.
48. Heckmatt J, Saunders C, Peters AM, Rose M, Hassan N, Thompson N, Cambridge G, Hyde SA, Dubowitz V. Cyclosporin in juvenile dermatomyositis. *Lancet* 1989; **i**:1063–6.
49. Dalakas MC, Illa I, Dambrosia JM, Soueidan SA, Stein DP, Otero C, Dinsmore ST, McCrosky S. A controlled trial of high-dose intravenous immune globulin infusions as treatment for dermatomyositis. *N Engl J Med* 1993; **329**:1993–2000.
50. Lang BA, Laxer RM, Murphy G, Silverman ED, Roifman CM. Treatment of dermatomyositis with intravenous immunoglobulin. *Am J Med* 1991; **91**:169–72.
51. Sansome A, Dubowitz V. Intravenous immunoglobulin in juvenile dermatomyositis – four year review of nine cases. *Arch Dis Child* 1995; **72**:25–8.
52. Collet E, Dalac S, Maerens B, Courtois JM, Izac M, Lambert D. Juvenile dermatomyositis – treatment with intravenous gammaglobulin. *Br J Derm* 1994; **130**:231–4.
53. Roifman CM, Schaffer FM, Wachsmuth SE, Murphy G, Gelfand EW. Reversal of chronic polymyositis following intravenous immune serum globulin therapy. *J Am Med Assoc* 1987; **258**:513–15.
54. Isenberg DA, Horsfall AC. Systemic lupus erythematosus-adult-onset. In: *Oxford Textbook of Rheumatology* (Maddison P, Isenberg D, Woo P, Glass D, eds.). Oxford University Press: Oxford, 1993:733–56.
55. Esdaile JM, Mackenzie ML, Kashgarian M, Hayslett JP. The benefit of early treatment with immunosuppressive agents in lupus nephritis. *J Rheum* 1994; **21**:2046–51.
56. Lehman TAJ. A practical guide to systemic lupus erythematosus. *Pediatr Clin North Am* 1995; **42**:1223–38.
57. Silverman ED, Eddy A. Systemic lupus erythematosus in childhood and adolescence. In: *Oxford Textbook of Rheumatology* (Maddison P, Isenberg D, Woo P, Glass D, eds.). Oxford University Press: Oxford, 1993:756–56.
58. Lehman TAJ. Cyclophosphamide for childhood SLE-A long-term success. *Arthritis Rheum* 1995; **38**:S363.
59. Walz LeBlanc BAE, Dagenais P, Urowitz MB, Gladman DD. Methotrexate in systemic lupus erythematosus. *J Rheum* 1994; **21**:733–36.
60. Wilson K, Abeles M. A 2 year, open-ended trial of methotrexate in systemic lupus erythematosus. *J Rheum* 1994; **21**:1674–7.
61. Abud-Mendoza C, Sturbaum A, Vazquez-Compean R, Gonzalez-Amaro R. Methotrexate therapy in childhood systemic lupus erythematosus. *J Rheum* 1993; **20**:731–3.

Index